THE ELEMENTS OF PRACTICAL PSYCHO-ANALYSIS

Founded by C. K. Ogden

The International Library of Psychology

PSYCHOANALYSIS
In 28 Volumes

THE ELEMENTS OF PRACTICAL PSYCHO-ANALYSIS

PAUL BOUSFIELD

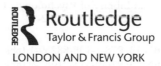

Routledge
Taylor & Francis Group
LONDON AND NEW YORK

First published in 1922
by Routledge, Trench, Trubner & Co., Ltd.
2 Park Square, Milton Park, Abingdon, Oxfordshire OX14 4RN
711 Third Avenue, New York, NY 10017

First issued in paperback 2014

Routledge is an imprint of the Taylor and Francis Group, an informa business

British Library Cataloguing in Publication Data
A CIP catalogue record for this book
is available from the British Library

The Elements of Practical Psycho-Analysis
ISBN 0415-21082-8
Psychoanalysis: 28 Volumes
ISBN 0415-21132-8
The International Library of Psychology: 204 Volumes
ISBN 0415-19132-7

ISBN 13: 978-1-138-88259-1 (pbk)
ISBN 13: 978-0-415-21082-9 (hbk)

PREFACE

THE object of this work is to give an account
of the theory, technique, and scope of psycho-
analysis, in such a form that its essentials may
readily be understood by the student or
practitioner without previous systematic reading
in psychology and psychotherapy.

At present should anyone wish to study the
subject, even if only to grasp its general import,
it is necessary for him to read not one, but
several, large volumes on the matter, each of
which will give him some information, but each
of which presupposes that the reader has
already mastered essential details in the course
of previous reading. Added to this the terminology in use is of a highly technical nature,
and to the beginner who has to refer continuously
to a dictionary (which often dues not contain the
word required) this is very disconcerting, and
frequently the reader is left with vague and
mistaken notions. A large number of medical
men have discussed this matter with me, and
have explained to me how difficult they have
found it to understand even the elements of the

subject, and as a result I feel that there is need of a concise and simple work on it which at the same time shall avoid as far as possible technical and foreign terms. It is this object that I have striven after in the present work. With regard to terminology, I have attempted to use ordinary English words whereever possible, but for the use of those who propose to read other works on the subject I have included a glossary of the technical terms in common use.

In one or two of the early examples of the mechanism of formation of special characteristics of the Psychoneuroses I have either invented simple typical cases or taken the liberty of modifying the details of slightly more complex cases, so that the ideas underlying them shall be perfectly plain to those who have not previously studied the subject ; while throughout the earlier chapters on the unconscious mind I have limited my choice for the same reason to a few quite simple ideas and examples, although more complicated material might sometimes have conveyed greater proof of the accuracy of certain theories. It must be understood that these examples are not cited as ⁂ proofs of the theories given ; such proof may be taken as having been demonstrated in many other larger works, and I have merely given examples to demonstrate these theories in a concise and elementary manner.

As probably most readers know, Freud is the originator of the technique and theory of the psychoanalytic system ; nevertheless, there are some points in his teaching which many regard as dogmatic and unproven, and a few of these points I shall mention shortly in the text. Some persons are very apt to take for granted that the whole work of a great pioneer is accurate and final, and this is dangerous if we are to progress and find further truth ; for even the greatest of scientists occasionally finds evidence which does not fit in with his theories and which therefore he tends to ignore or unconsciously to falsify, so as to fit it in with his other ideas. The three notable subjects on which I consider Freud's evidence to be insufficient are :—firstly, in his theory of *complete* determinism as opposed to Free Will ; secondly, in his statement that *all* Dreams have the same causative factors ; and thirdly, in his theory that sexual desire is the fundamental desire underlying *all* other desires and emotions. It will be seen, however, that this does not in any way affect our acceptance of his technique, his theory of dreams in the great majority of cases, and his theory of the etiology of most of the neuroses and psychoneuroses. To him must always be given the credit of having discovered what will probably prove to be one of the most significant factors in the future development of the human race. The last chapter of this book is devoted to a discussion illustrating possible ways in which psycho-analysis will become a factor, not merely in curing the neurosis of a patient, but also in discovering deleterious matter in the mental attitudes of the race as a whole, and by such discoveries enable us gradually to reform them.

PAUL BOUSFIELD.

7, Harley Street, W.
January, 1920

GLOSSARY

Abasia. Inability to walk.

Abreaction. The process of working off the emotion arising out of an unpleasant experience by living through the incident again.

Affect. Feeling. The energy belonging to emotion. The unit of psychic energy attached to an idea.

Agoraphobia. Morbid fear of open spaces.

Algolagnia. Abnormal activity of sexual impulse, with a desire for experiencing or causing pain. Includes Sadism and Masochism.

Allo-erotism. Erotic feelings of any kind directed towards another person (of either sex).

Ambivalence. The coexistence of opposed feelings.

Amnesia. A definite complete loss of memory for a given period or event.

Anæsthesia. Loss of physical sensation.

Anal-eroticism. Erotic emotions caused by stimulation of the anal regions.

Aphonia. Inability to speak.

Astasia. Inability to stand.

Auto-erotism. Erotic feelings of any kind generated in and directed towards oneself.

Bi-sexual. (1). Pertaining to, or containing, the characteristics of both sexes, whether physically or mentally. (2). Having erotic feelings for members of both sexes.

Catharsis. A mental purging brought about by bringing unpleasant thoughts or experiences to the surface : *cf.* Abreaction.

Censor. The repressing force in the mind which tends to prevent the unpleasant from becoming conscious.

Cloacal Erotism. Erotic emotions caused by stimulating any of those parts originally enclosed in the cloaca, *e.g.*, anus, vagina, urethra.

Cloaca Theory. The infantile belief concerning birth per rectum.

Claustrophobia. Morbid fear of enclosed spaces.

Coitus interruptus. The withdrawal of the male organ before the orgasm, so that emission takes place outside.

Coitus reservatus. Delayed coitus, in which one of the parties deliberately holds back the orgasm, or in which orgasm does not take place.

Complex. A system or group of ideas bearing upon one central idea, the whole or a part of which system is repressed together with its emotional tone.

Condensation. The unconscious fusion of several ideas, so as to form one composite whole, *e.g.*, a composite photograph is one final portrait though composed of many super-imposed original photographs.

Constellation. Any system, or group, of ideas not repressed.

Conversion. The expression of repressed (unpleasant) emotional ideas by means of a physical manifestation.

Coprophilia. Interest in the products of excretion.

Displacement. The transference of psychic energy or feeling from one idea to another but without alteration in the original emotional tone : *cf.* Sublimation.

Erogenous Zone. Any special area of the body which may, when stimulated, give rise to erotic emotions.

Euphoria. A feeling of well-being.

Exhibitionism. Erotic gratification in exhibiting the genital organs or some other erogenous zone.

Fetishism. Erotic gratification in connection with a part only of the loved object's clothing, *e.g.*, a handkerchief or glove.

Hetero-erotism. See Allo-erotism.

Hetero-sexuality. Erotic desires towards one of the opposite sex (the normal adult condition).

Homo-sexuality. Erotic desires towards one of the same sex (an infantile or primitive condition, which may persist into adult life).

Idiogamist. A man potent with only one particular woman (or limited type of women) and impotent with all others.

Incest. A sexual act with, or erotic desires towards, a near relative.

Introjection. The absorbtion of external events into oneself, so that one reacts to these events as though they took place in or were part of one's own self.

Libido. Erotic desire : used vaguely by some writers to include the whole " life desire " or the " psychic energy " entailed in gratifying it ; and used by others in a much more restricted sense, the degree of which varies with the writer.

Masochism. Sexual perversion, with enjoyment of being cruelly treated.

Masturbation. The auto-erotic manipulation of one's own reproductive organs for the purpose of procuring a sexual orgasm.

Narcissism. Self-worship. Probably pre-natal in origin, and for a short period non-sexual. It soon, however, attaches itself to the auto-erotic complexes and constellations.

Nosophobia. Fear of disease.

Oral Erotism. Erotic emotions caused by stimulation of the mouth or lips.

Projection. Ascribing one's own inner complexes to other persons, unconsciously throwing upon the outer world and ascribing to it the working of one's own mind.

Rationalization. The invention of reasons for ideas or actions when the real motive is not recognised consciously.

Regression. Psychic reversion to an earlier or more primitive type of mental life, signalized by more primitive forms of energic expression (generally erotic).

Repression. Preventing unpleasant ideas and conflicts from becoming conscious, or forcing such from the conscious content of the mind if they had already become conscious.

Resistance. The obstructive force tending to keep unpleasant material repressed and refusing to allow such material to enter the conscious mind. " The Censor."

Sadism. The erotic enjoyment of causing pain, mental or physical : *cf.* Masochism.

Sublimation. The transference of erotic energy from a sexual to a non-sexual objective, the latter being useful socially. It differs from Displacement in that the latter merely transfers erotic energy from one sexual objective to another sexual objective which is less obvious to the conscious mind as being sexual.

Transference. The act of transfering (displacing) psychic energy from one idea to another. In the case of analysis, from one person to the psychoanalyst.

Trauma. Injury, psychic or physical.

Voyeur. Erotic gratification in looking at the genital organs or some other erogenous zone.

Zöophilia Eroticism. Erotic gratification in touching, petting, etc., animals.

Elements of Practical Psycho-Analysis

CHAPTER I

THE UNCONSCIOUS MIND

BEFORE defining psycho-analysis or discussing its technique, it is essential that we should have a clear conception of the mind as regards its unconscious elements, and the functions of these with reference to ideas, desires and emotions.

Freud and other psychologists have divided the mind into several constituents : conscious, fore-conscious, subconscious, unconscious and other terms are frequently met with, but for our purpose a simple division into *conscious* and *unconscious* will suffice. The CONSCIOUS MIND needs but little discussion here. It is that part of the mind which knows and feels and reasons in the immediate present, and which defines itself sufficiently for elementary purposes : it is conscious.

The UNCONSCIOUS MIND is, however, more elusive, and requires a good deal of consideration. In the first place, it is the storehouse of facts and ideas—in other words, *mem-*

ory. At any given moment we have in our conscious mind very few memories ; we are not aware of the vast number of experiences through which we have passed during our lives. We know, however, that by turning our attention in the desired direction, we can find and bring to consciousness a very great number of these memories. Most of the time, however, it is obvious that we are certainly not conscious of them. These memories of the past may be said to be " stored " in the unconscious part of the mind.

This brings us to the point that, while we can, by making the requisite effort bring into the conscious mind many memories, and while other past facts are only brought to mind by some chance association with external stimuli, there are yet other experiences which we have totally forgotten, and which are never revived as conscious memories.

Let us consider examples of these types of memory and trace some of the underlying causes.

In the first place, one can remember with very little effort with whom one dined last Saturday evening. The event is what is commonly termed " still fresh in the memory." One has a good deal more difficulty in remembering, however, which was the last play one witnessed at a theatre. The event took place some weeks ago, and one has been to several theatres in the last few months. My conscious method of remembering my last visit to the theatre is as follows. I try to remember firstly when it occurred, secondly with whom I went, thirdly whether I dined at home that evening, fourthly what work I was doing at that period and how I could possibly have managed to find time for a theatre, since I was particularly busy about that period, and so forth. In other words, one gropes round for a clue, *i.e.*, an *association* connected with it. Perhaps my last thought about work is that which gives me my association—or rather, train of associations; it runs thus: "Certainly I was very busy, but now I remember one of my patients could not come to see me; he telephoned to me; yes, and I telephoned to my brother and asked him to meet me at the club. We dined there and discussed our plans, and finally went to His Majesty's theatre to see 'Hamlet.'"

We see at once then that here our memory depends on finding some incident in association with the fact we are seeking, and following up that association with others. It may be that ones thoughts flow rapidly and that the result appears to "flash" into ones mind, but however this may be, the evidence tends to show that *all* memories depend upon such a train of associations. And these *associations bring into the conscious mind those facts which were previously hidden away in the unconscious mind.*

As an example of those memories which require an external stimulus to bring them into consciousness the following may be cited. I remember distinctly an advertisement for a certain tooth paste, but no amount of groping for associations enables me to locate the place where I saw it. By chance while I am walking down the road I see a model battleship in a shop window : at once there rushes to my mind the fact that next to the advertisement for the tooth paste was another one extolling a certain whiskey in which a battleship figured in the foreground. I further remember I discussed the scarcity of whiskey with a friend while we were travelling on the underground railway and had just got out at Oxford Circus. *That* was where I saw the advertisement in question.

Here we find that the train of association takes us right to our objective, once we find a starting point. We might in time have found one somewhere in the mind, instead of externally, but the event itself was trivial and we had no outstanding associations on which we could seize readily. The external stimulus, however, supplied the first association, and the memory quickly followed it into consciousness.

We now come to the third example. There are obviously some experiences which no ordinary method will bring into consciousness. If one were to be asked where one had dined on the 17th of March, 1901, it is extremely unlikely that one would be able to remember. The memory is apparently lost, and for ever. Nevertheless, did one happen to keep a detailed diary of one's doings, one might discover the hidden fact, and by the many associations in the diary actually *then* recall the fact.

Psycho-analysis shows us that by suitable technique we actually can recover memories far back in childhood, apparently buried for ever, when the right train of associations is tapped. Under hypnosis we can similarly call back memories with a detail and exactitude which is scarcely believable until it has been tested. Nothing is apparently really forgotten. Every word in a conversation which took place 20 years ago, may be readily and accurately brought to mind in some hypnotized subjects.

This now leads us to consider the various *reasons* why we should ever have lost the train of associations leading to these forgotten experiences. One reason we already know: an event was of no importance and only a trivial mental association was formed which in itself takes much seeking.

There are, however, other reasons why we lose our associations and forget events ; these we will now proceed to discuss.

We often forget things because either we do not like to remember them, or else they are associated with something which we do not like to remember. This is particularly the case with mental conflicts, which we refuse to solve consciously on the grounds that whatever solution we arrived at would be unpleasant.

This form of forgetting we term *repression.* The unpleasant memory and *associations which might call it to mind* are repressed from the conscious into the unconscious.

Darwin writes in his autobiography :

" I had, during many years, followed a golden rule, namely, that whenever a published fact, a new observation or thought came across me, which was opposed to my general results, to make a memorandum of it without fail and at once ; for I had found by experience that such facts and thoughts were far more apt to escape from the memory than favourable ones."

In these cases of forgetting—*i.e.,* by repression, there is always a conflict between the *conscious* will and the *unconscious* counter-will. We shall see later that the unconscious will is a very real factor.

The conscious will feebly tries to remember, while the unconscious counter-will emphatically says : " This is unpleasant ; it shall not be remembered." An excellent example is related by Maeder. A house surgeon had a business appointment in town, but he was not allowed to leave the hospital until his chief, who was out to dinner, should return later in the evening. As his appointment in town was important he decided to brave the anger of his chief and go into town. When he returned later he found to his astonishment that he had left the light in his room burning—a thing he had never done before, although he had occupied that room for two years. On thinking the matter over he soon realized why he had done this. His chief in passing the window to his own house would see the light burning and imagine that his house surgeon was within. The unconscious mind had determined that the turning out of the light should be forgotten (repressed).

Examples in everyday life are very common. We mislay bills very readily : rarely do we mislay a cheque. We forget to post letters entrusted to us against our will ; but we do not forget to post our own love letters.

An example from my own experience will

illustrate a common type of this repression. I had to attend a lecture on Psychotherapy given by a man with whose views I totally disagreed, and which I did not wish to attend, but felt compelled to do in an official capacity. First of all I wrote the time of the lecture in my engagement book a week late. On discovering this I omitted for a moment to rectify it, and when I eventually did so, I put it down for Tuesday instead of Thursday. Later, on being asked by several friends on which day the lecture was, I told them that it was on Tuesday instead of Thursday (thus unconsciously trying to make them also miss the lecture). Finally I made an appointment for a patient at the real time appointed for the lecture. Now I had attended regularly most of the lectures at the institution in question and had generally looked forward to them. It was only in the case of this one lecture, which I consciously disliked yet had decided to attend, that my unconscious counter-will attempted time after time to prevent my so doing.

The examples of the repression of memory so far given apply only to small and comparatively unimportant matters, but the same principles hold good in very important or outstanding features of life. Very many patients suffering from " shell shock " and other nervous diseases of the war exhibit lapses of memory comprising whole weeks or months of their service on the one hand or some unutterably horrible or disgusting incident on the other hand—such matters as one would expect to be indelibly impressed upon the mind. And I have had patients who had completely forgotten the whole of their past lives.

One such patient of mine had completely forgotten how his two great friends had come by their death, although he was standing near them at the time and saw the shell explode which had killed them both. One of his friends had had the whole of the back of his head blown away, and the other his abdomen ripped open. This horrible event was completely repressed from conscious memory *as well as associations connected with the event which might have led to its remembrance*. A complete small section of his life was " split off from consciousness " and forgotten (amnesia). These memories were brought back gradually by the method of free association practised in psycho-analysis. I will try and illustrate by a simple example how this " splitting of consciousness " or *dissociation* might take place.

If I write down a list of eight words each absolutely unconnected with one another, the average reader will find it very lifficult after

reading the list through once to remember the
words in their written order, and to repeat the
list either backwards or forwards, for example :

>kettle
>bluebell
>writing-desk
>engine
>flower-pot
>poultice
>table
>poker

There is no *association* between each word, and
one word does not tend to bring the next into
consciousness.

If, however, I use a list of words each one of
which is associated with the next in some
definite manner it will be found comparatively
easy to repeat that list either backwards or
forwards after once reading it :—

>ink
>black
>mourning
>death
>ghost
>Hamlet
>Shakespeare
>Bacon

There is in this list some definite association
between each word, and as one word is spoken

it brings up automatically and with little effort
the next word out of the unconscious. Suppose
now the memories of "death" and "ghost" to be
unpleasant—that we wish to repress the ideas.
We may *unconsciously* falsify our association at
the word "mourning" and thus leave out
one letter and substitute the word "morning."
This might be done in several ways : either
by means of a play on words we might inter-
polate the word "morning" thus :

        ink
        black
        mourning
        morning

or by adding an extra association, thus :

        ink
        black
        night
        morning

In either case the associations of "morning"
are so absolutely different from those of "mourning" that the rest of the words are no longer
called into consciousness. We have *dissociated*
them. They are now *repressed*.

*A repressed group or constellation of ideas is
technically known as a Complex.*

Extreme cases of dissociation have been
known to bring about what is known as " dual
personalities," in which one person appears to

live two completely separate lives with two quite dissimilar sets of characteristics and memories An excellent example of this is given by R. L. Stevenson in " Dr. Jekyll and Mr. Hyde." The different characteristics of the two personalities in all such cases are accounted for by the fact that in one case the *conscious* will is in the ascendency, and in the other the *unconscious* counter-will. (The unconscious will is primarily selfish, self-seeking and desirous of defending the person from unpleasantness as far as possible. We shall discuss this, however, at a later period).

The unconscious mind, however, has far more functions than that of conserving memories, or of falsifying or repressing them. In the examples given we can observe that not only have memories been repressed unconsciously, but that this unconscious process has involved the factors of *will, intellect, desire* and *emotion.* Apart from exercising these functions, however, the unconscious mind is capable of working in some respects more efficiently than the conscious mind. It can reason clearly, it can control to some extent the physiological functions of the body, it can carry out complicated automatic actions known as " habits,": it can to some extent register the thoughts of others by a " sixth sense," as yet but little understood, the process being known as telepathy.

As examples of unconscious reasoning we already have the case of the house surgeon who omitted to turn out the light in his room. But this, though cunning reasoning, was not on a very high level. A friend of mine once told me that he had spent several days in trying to work out a chess problem without success. One morning he woke up with a picture in his mind of the exact moves which he must make. He had solved the problem in his sleep unconsciously, and with no recollection on waking of any conscious effort at reaching this solution. In my own experience as a schoolboy, I failed to solve a problem of Euclid during an examination. On the morning afterwards the solution flashed through my brain suddenly as I lay in bed. Whether I had solved this in my sleep, or whether it was solved in bed as I lay awake, I am not prepared to say, but this much is quite certain—I made no conscious effort at reasoning; my mind merely wandered lazily in the direction of the previous day's failure, and almost instantaneously the right solution appeared without an effort. No doubt many readers will have experienced similar examples of unconscious reasoning of this type.

As regards the unconscious control of physical functions a well known example is the fact that on watching somebody suck a lemon our own mouths will " water." Suggestion, whether under hypnosis or not, can cause physiological action to be inhibited or increased. As a student I once gave a fellow student who suffered from constipation two pills made of bread, assuring him that they were composed of a very powerful aperient. He took them gratefully, suffered a good deal of colic, and they acted as I had suggested. I may add that my friend was readily hypnotisable and a good recipient of " suggestion." This does not, however, detract from the fact that, *giving no further conscious thought to the matter*, his unconscious mind controlled the physiological action of his intestines. Many wonderful cures by means of patent medicines obviously take place in a similar manner. I give only one or two simple instances of these various functions of the unconscious mind, because in this chapter I wish merely to demonstrate shortly its scope and widespread power. We shall then more clearly apprehend in future chapters the more complex mechanisms involved in the neuroses and psychoneuroses.

Referring now to complex actions, including those which come within the term " habit," one need only cite as an example the playing of an accomplished pianist. He reads the music

in front of him consciously, but the translation
of this through the brain and into the fingers
so as to produce a series of extremely rapid and
complicated movements on the keyboard of
the piano is quite unconscious. He does not
look at the keys of the piano ; he does not think,
" With which finger shall I play this note, or
that ? " The *sorting out* of the fingering and
adaptation of it to the keys as he reads a new
piece of music is something which takes place
entirely in his unconscious mind.

I have mentioned the subject of thought-
transference or telepathy as one of the functions
of the unconscious mind. I have done so not
because it is of very much importance, but
because Freud and other writers ignore its
existence, and because I have had definite
proof that it occupies a place, though at present
a small one, in the list of functions of the unconscious mind, and thus modifies slightly one
or two of the more dogmatic statements of
these writers on points to be discussed in a
future chapter. I refer to the classification of
dreams and hallucinations.

I am fortunate in possessing a friend who
has developed telepathic powers to a considerable degree, and from boyhood upwards, I and
my relatives have had every opportunity of
testing his powers under our own conditions.

We have grown to look upon his powers as something more or less ordinary, and indeed have devised a new drawing-room game based upon them. I wish to give here one or two of the experiments which have taken place, not once only but very many times. In the following paragraphs I refer to him as Mr. X.

Mr. X is sent into an adjoining room quite out of earshot, while we then decide upon some trivial action which he shall perform, such as picking up the poker and carrying it across the room and presenting it to Mrs. B. Mr. X, blindfolded, is now called into the room. Nobody touches him. Everyone sits perfectly quiet, no sound or word of any kind is spoken. Those sitting in the room now " will " his *movements, i.e.,* first that he shall walk to the right spot where lies the poker, then that he shall stoop, then stretch out his arm in the right direction, and so forth. As a rule, with very little hesitation the whole performance is gone through without a hitch. Such experiments, however, must be fairly simple in character ; thus, while we can make Mr. X walk to the piano, open it and sit down, we have never succeeded in conveying to his mind a particular tune which we wish him to play. During these experiments he describes his own part as consisting in " making his mind a blank " and moving as if under compulsion. As the sitters are not always the same on all occasions there is no possibility of any system of signs.

A variant of this experiment is as follows: two groups of persons are formed. One group settles upon one set of actions, say, that Mr. X shall take the poker and present it to Mrs. B. The other group selects a different set of actions —perhaps that he shall remove a hairpin from the head of Mrs. C and place it on a given chair. When Mr. X comes in a contest thus takes place. Perhaps, after a pause, the concentrated efforts of the first group succeed in getting him to pick up the poker. There may be then a feeling of triumph and relief in that group, with a consequent momentary relaxation of concentration. Immediately this takes place Mr. X will perform part of the plan formed by the second group; he will rush to the chair and place the poker on the chair where the hairpin should have been placed. A variety of similar experiments have taken place.

Perhaps the most convincing and at the same time one of the simplest experiments is as follows, and it is one which absolutely prevents any trickery whatsoever.

Mr. X sits in a chair with his back to me (or any other suitable person); he is at one side of a room and I am at the other. There need be no other person in the room. I take a pack of cards, shuffle it, look at one card, concentrate my mind upon it, and say simply the one word " Now ! " Mr. X at the other side of the room, with his back to me (or blind-folded) names the card in detail, thus, " Queen of Hearts." And so we proceeded through the whole pack. The only word spoken is " Now ! " Mr. X never gets all the cards right ; frequently there are mistakes, but the majority of the cards are named correctly. To anyone who has performed such experiments as these, time after time, there can be no doubt about the existence of telepathy, and that it merits a place in the functions of the unconscious mind. One can merely state that there is a sixth sense —the telepathic sense—but its exact method of action is as yet veiled from us. This aspect of the unconscious mind will, however, not enter materially into our work of psycho-analysis. It is mentioned here merely to convey a more complete idea of the complex processes which are continually taking place uncon-sciously within us.

In all the examples I have hitherto given of unconscious activity it will be noticed that nothing of an unselfish nature is apparent. Two fundamental ruling instincts are con-stantly at work in our unconscious mind, as

they have been in the unconscious of our remote
ancestors right back to the simplest forms of
life. These are the instincts of self-preservation
and of propagation—the desire to preserve life
and to propagate the species. They are exhibited in every child from the tenderest years,
and persist into old age. The " purest minded "
of persons, who never gives a thought to sexual
matters, or the saint who welcomes martyrdom,
still possess these instincts and their various
modified desires, though these may be totally
repressed, or otherwise disguised, as we shall
see in later chapters. As we proceed with our
investigations we shall find that in cases where
the unconscious will or desires are discoverable,
self-centred motives are for the most part
present. The unconscious mind, in other words,
is largely ego-centric. It attempts continuously
to defend the self, or to obtain pleasures, gratify
desires, get rid of unpleasant conflicts, etc.
The unconscious mind is primitive in its origin
and often brutal. Even in the greatest saint
on earth does this hold good : if we analyse his
unconscious acts we shall discover the many
complex ego-centric motives.

SUMMARY.

1. *In the unconscious mind will, intelligence,
desire and some other attributes of the*

      conscious mind are developed in a high degree.

2.   *The unconscious mind is the seat of memory, habit and other functions not present at all in the conscious mind.*

3.   *Insoluble and unpleasant mental conflicts, ideas and desires may become repressed and completely forgotten, together with associations which might tend to revive them.*

4.   *Memories long forgotten or repressed may be brought into the conscious mind again by finding suitable associations.*

5.   *The unconscious mind conflicts frequently with the conscious mind, and where the unconscious will (counter-will) is stronger than the conscious will, memories, resolutions and unpleasant material may be repressed from the conscious into the unconscious and unconscious desires may be satisfied.*

6.   *The unconscious mind is always to a great degree primitive and self-centred.*

CHAPTER II

DESIRES AND PSYCHIC ENERGY

A LARGE part of every one's life is devoted to wishing and attempting to gratify wishes. Desire of one kind or another rules the major portion of our time, and these desires may be very varied in character. The dipsomaniac is constantly desiring alcohol, the scientist is desiring discovery. If his work be interrupted by household matters, he desires ardently to get back to his work. Some women desire " pretty " clothes, others desire a beautiful home. One desires rest, another gaiety and excitement. We shall find on analysis that the *energy* behind these desires can for the most part be traced to the two primitive instincts mentioned in the last chapter—namely, self-preservation and self-propagation, or perhaps it would be more accurate to say to the ultimate instinct of *vital continuity*.

Let us take an example. A man becomes devoted to the game of tennis, and much physical energy is expended in playing the game, but behind this much mental or psychic energy is also expended. The *desire* to play, if there were no *energy behind that desire*, would avail nothing. There must be sufficient force to cause the man *to act*, seize his racquet and balls and overcome his physical inertia throughout a hot afternoon. Let us just examine this in a purely superficial manner for the moment. One of the constantly recurring expressions we hear is, " I must get some exercise ! " or, " I need more exercise ! " Why is this ? Exercise is required to keep us in health. Health is necessary to the prolongation of life. Ultimately, then, many people have the instinct of *self-preservation*, to some extent at any rate, behind their desire to play tennis. There is, however, another unconscious motive. It is well known that sports are commonly encouraged at school, at any rate to some extent, because experience shows that morbid sexuality is less in those who expend their energy in the excitement and emotion of sports than in those who are averse from outdoor games.

Now sexual desire is one of the forms of desire we are taught to repress from childhood upwards, but though we may often very successfully repress conflicts connected with this desire into the unconscious *yet the energy belonging to this desire is still present, and must find some outlet for its discharge.* Tennis, with its elements of *excitement*, mental and physical, as well as possibly its element of rhythmic motion, furnishes to some extent this outlet. It is the same with other forms of sport. Hence the repression of sexual desire may lead to a desire to expend the energy in some other exciting manner. Thus our tennis player may have much that is ultimately concerned with both self-preservation and self-propagation behind his desire to play tennis.

Such a transference of psychic energy from an undesirable to a desirable form of discharge is known as *sublimation*. Sport is not the only method of sublimation, however ; religion, art, music, mathematics, science, etc., all perform a similar function, while in the opposite direction alcoholism, drug-taking, hysterias and psychoneuroses of various kinds may act as an outlet for such repressed energy of desire on a lower plane, yet still in such a manner that prevents the crude instincts and their ensuing mental conflicts from entering too often or too forcibly into the conscious mind. The matter is not nearly so simple as one might imagine from the above paragraphs. At present I am only attempting to give a general idea of it ; we shall later find the mechanism behind the changing forms of " energy of desire " to be of a somewhat complex nature.

This leads us to consider the term, " energy of desire."   " Psychic energy " is another name which we can give to it : some have called it " mental energy."

It will aid our conception of this mental or psychic energy if we first consider for a moment physical energy.

We know as regards physical energy that there are not several kinds of energy, but merely several manifestations of it, and that it may be changed from one form of manifestation to another, but that still the sum total of the original energy remains without addition or loss.

Thus there is a given amount of energy stored in a ton of coal   This energy can manifest itself as *heat* in the furnace and boiler. By means of an engine we can change the manifestation into that of *motion*, then with a dynamo to *electricity ;* the electricity we can again change into *light*, or back into *heat* or *motion*.   There is *one* energy, but by suitable means we can turn it to different uses, and give different manifestations of it.   Owing, however, to the imperfection of our boiler, machinery, etc., we never transform the *whole* of our energy into another form.   In transforming heat into electricity there is always some heat wasted ; it is not destroyed, but it remains as heat for a time, and is absorbed by surrounding objects. A complete transference of energy does not take place, and the less efficient the machinery the less efficient is the transference.

Now evidence tends to show a considerable analogy between psychic and physical energy. In all probability there is only one ultimate psychic energy, which, like physical energy, can be directed into different channels. Thus the energy of erotic desire can be directed to a large extent into the energy of desire for music, religion, science or sport ; or the energy of the desire for sport may be changed into the energy of desire for mental exercise, such as chess, mathematics or science. For example, an individual feels " restless " : he then desires to play tennis ; the afternoon is wet ; he plays chess instead. His psychic energy has been diverted from one channel into another with its accompanying excitement and satisfaction of desire ; with its final feeling of fatigue and repletion.

Psychic energy, like physical energy, can never be entirely diverted from one channel to another. There is always some, often a large quantity, which is not altered in character. The amount of this depends largely on the person concerned, just as the amount of physical energy, changed from one form to another depends on the efficiency of the engine or machinery.

This possibility of transference of energy of desire from one form to another is of the utmost importance to the psycho-analyst. By the technique of psycho-analysis the energy of repressed desires is first freed from deleterious, and then transferred to legitimate objectives. The energy behind the desires of the alcoholic or drug-taker may, under suitable conditions, be transferred to energy of higher types of desire, with more suitable outlets. These processes are known as *transference displacement* and *sublimation* respectively.

It may be taken that every mind has a given amount of psychic energy which *must* find somewhere its suitable outlet in satisfying desire.

We may here take the opportunity of remarking that the efficiency or lack of efficiency demonstrated in different individuals in their attempts to transfer the energy of desire from a lower to a higher channel depends not only on heredity and constitutional circumstances but to an extraordinary degree on the individual's environment and the actions of the parents in the first three or four years of his life. The reason why seemingly excellent parents produce sometimes execrable progeny becomes clearer under psycho-analysis. The over-strict parent produces one type of inefficient children, the parent who spoils produces other inefficient types. The nurse, the nursery, the casual visitor, the trivial conversations, the unconsidered sights and experiences, all have a terrific influence in the first few years of the child's life. Parents do not realize that conventional or arbitrary methods of education, whether in one direction or another, are not going to effect the results they expected. The primitive unconscious mind of the child understands and absorbs in a manner that civilised man does not recognise. The bad father may by accident or *neglect* produce an excellent child —the good father with all his designs may produce a bad one. This is not an attempt to shew that as the child grows up all its actions are dependent on the early environment ; merely that we can never compare the good or bad in individuals ; that an apparent failure, owing to his inefficiency of powers of sublimation, may yet be devoting more energy to ascent than the successful saint whose early environment made for efficient transference of energy of desire. Some of the commonest of errors made by well-meaning parents will come to light at a later period. *They teach their children to repress erotic and other desires but they omit*

*to assist the development of that sublimation which
is absolutely essential at the same time.*

The word *libido* is often used by psycho-
analysts instead of the words " energy of
desire." The very different meanings applied
to it, however, seem to me to make the word
libido an unsuitable one to use. The Freudian
school mean by *libido* the energy of all forms
of sexual desire, in its broadest sense ; other
authorities use it to designate *all* forms of
psychic energy, and there are yet others who
place it somewhere between the two. Hence
in this book I shall avoid the use of the term ;
it is, however, necessary for persons who intend
to read other works on psycho-analysis to have
some idea of what meaning different writers
attach to the word *libido*.

Having pointed out that psychic energy
appears to be of one kind only, though manifesting itself in different ways, the question
arises, what is its fundamental and primitive
source ?

Freud holds, as the result of far reaching
studies that the energy of sexual desire is at
the root of practically all other forms, even in
infancy. His conclusions follow upon years of
careful research ; he sees in the suckling of an
infant at the mother's breast the earliest form
of sexual satisfaction in the infant. The desire,

the evident pleasure, followed by complete
satiety, flushing and sleep he compares with
the fulfilment ot normal sexual intercourse of
later life. He shows that the breast and mouth,
as well as the arms, eyes, nose and various parts
of the skin and the reproductive organs themselves are all erotic zones ; that is, that they
have some kind of sexual significance in early
life which often persists in various people in a
modified form after puberty. But with all the
evidence which he adduces I do not consider
that he has proved the nutritional desire of
infancy to be an early and undifferentiated part
of sexual desire.

We mentioned previously two great primitive instincts—the desire for self-preservation
and the desire for self-propagation or continuance of the species (erotic desire). The two
are no doubt very intimately connected and
probably both are derived from a still more
primitive and undifferentiated " life " desire.*
But there is certainly evidence to show that
the nutritional instinct is nearer that of self-
preservation than of sexual desire, for all its
superficial resemblances.

Let us take as an example one of the most
primitive life histories possible—that of the

---

*This " life desire " I have called " the instinct of vital con-
tinuity " in other parts of this work, as representing the ultimate
instinct in the most primitive and undifferentiated forms of life.

amœba. The young amœba spends its energy solely in growth and in acquiring food. As an individual it only has one sexual act of any kind in its life history, and that is at the end of its individual life, when its nucleus divides into two parts, and the amœba itself then follows suit, constituting two new young amœbæ. It is possible to argue that it begins its life with a sexual act of the parent amœba, and that all its life is devoted to preparing for a sexual act of its own, whereby the species shall be continued. But one may equally well argue that its chief energy is devoted to acquiring nourishment, and only when it finds its powers of assimilation failing does it then rest and perform its sexual act as a means of rejuvenescence, that it may once more get back to its pleasure of assimilating food.

On the face of it, the longest part of its life is devoted to *self-preservation* rather than to *self-propagation*, but the two are equally necessary to the continuance of the species. It surely would be better to describe the energy of both as alternating manifestations of an instinct of vital continuity, rather than to ascribe the nutritional element as a form of the sexual element. Indeed, it would appear to be more logical to speak of the sexual element in any individual as being one of the manifestations of the instinct of self-preservation, and of assuming even that it may develop later out of nutritional processes, rather than stating that the infantile nutritional process is a manifestation of infantile sexual desire.

I am not disputing Freud's fact that sexual desires begin to manifest themselves in infancy, but that all other manifestations of desire should be reduced to a sexual basis. Many of his disciples reduce all form of *fear* to a sexual basis—*i.e.*, the fear of death is an unconscious fear that one will no longer be able to continue to propagate the species by sexuality. It seems more reasonable to suppose that such fear is a result of the unconscious instinct of vital continuity, and that in itself it is a reaction against the destruction of life rather than of the nerve power to reproduce the species. The whole is greater than the part.

SUMMARY

1. *Life activity is chiefly composed of various desires and the effort to gratify desires.*
2. *Most desires can be traced ultimately to the primitive desire to continue and preserve life (the instinct of vital continuity).*
3. *To attain any desire we must use a form of energy which we term psychic or mental energy.*

4. *Psychic energy, like physical energy, appears to be of one kind only, though it may, like physical energy have many forms of manifestation.*

5. *Like physical energy, one form of psychic energy can be transformed into another form, but never completely—always some remains in the original form. The amount unchanged depends on the efficiency of the particular personal machinery.*

6. *The energy of sexual desire is constantly repressed, but it must and will find an outlet somewhere, if in another form.*

CHAPTER III

THE EVOLUTION OF EROTIC DESIRE

NOTE.—*I have not endeavoured to prove the conclusions drawn in this chapter. The proof involves in itself enough work to fill several volumes, and consists largely of the results of psycho-analytic research. I have merely tried to give a clear conception of the facts by comparative means, by examples taken in different forms of primitive life, many of which are known to everyone to persist in the adult life of abnormal individuals. I have tried to show the steps of psychic evolution by simple references to comparative psychology in much the same way that one demonstrates to a student human anatomical values by means of comparative anatomy. Those readers who wish to see more of the evidence proving the facts given in this chapter should read Freud's " Three Contributions to the Theory of Sex " ; also his " Selected Papers on Hysteria and other Psychoneuroses," and his " Interpretation of Dreams " ; Pfister's " Psycho-analytic*

33

Method " ; Imry's different works and Brill's work, all contribute their evidence to the whole. In a short text book it is impossible of course to give full proof of all the facts arrived at by previous workers.

Many will wonder why we should discuss sexuality at such length, having expressed the opinion that Freud has dogmatised too freely in reducing every desire to this ultimate basis. We shall attempt in a few words to show the reason of this, before proceeding with our consideration of sexual evolution.

We have seen that our Instinct for Vital Continuity expresses itself in the two subsidiary instincts of self-preservation and self-propagation.

Now we shall find that the manifestations of the energy behind these instincts overlap considerably ; that what is in the first place a means of self-preservation may afterwards become also an important factor in self-propagation ; that at different times the same expression of energy may subserve both purposes.

But whereas the meaning of energy displayed may be clear when considered in conjunction with self-preservation, it is far from clear when the statement is first made that it is a constituent of sexuality.

This, then, is one reason why the discussion of sexual evolution is of importance. A second, and very much more important reason is that desires and conflicts in connection with self-preservation are not repressed, and, the progress of civilization has made self-preservation a much less arduous task than in the days of our pre-human forefathers, and much of the energy once devoted to self-preservation is now freed and flows through erotic channels instead. This is especially the case in females and in those who do not have to grapple with the problem of " earning a living." On the other hand we are taught from childhood upwards to repress sexual desire and all thought connected with it ; and since, much of our energy that was previously used in self-preservation has now been freed from that channel and flows into the channel of self-propagation, this repression is rendered more difficult. Thus civilised conditions have constantly magnified the differentiation of sex artificially and have increased erotic energy by utilizing some of the energy of self-preservation, and having made this increase they then proceed to repress this energy —a course which is taken by no other animal under the sun. The result is that unless suitable sublimation takes place we have all kinds of psychoneuroses on the one hand, and perversions and "bad habits" of various kinds on the other hand. Hence we find it absolutely essential to any analysis of the unconscious to have a thorough understanding of the components of sexuality and the side channels into which their energy may turn.

The idea is commonly prevalent that sexual instincts consist of a strong impulse towards the other sex, which arises in the individual as puberty approaches. Nothing is further from the truth. The attraction to sexual connection between opposite sexes is merely a part of and a climax to many varied impulses arising at different periods from infancy onwards, and having aims quite apart from sexual connection with one of the opposite sex.

As our bodies repeat the stages of our evolution so also do our minds; and as our bodies still retain much that belongs to our earliest progenitors so also do our minds.

We spoke previously of the "sexuality" of the primitive amœba. It has no sex. It has no differentiated organs. The potentiality of reproduction *ad infinitum* exists within itself. It merely divides first its nucleus and then its whole self, becoming thus two new young individuals. The earliest type is thus monosexual and autosexual. Even as the type grows more complex under the process of evolution we find this autosexuality persisting along with bisexuality. A little higher in the evolutionary scale we find the paramoecium. At one time in its life it will divide first its nucleus and then itself also (an autosexual act) as in the case of the amœba. At another time it will perform an elementary sexual act by coming ventrally together with another paramoecium, and having split its nucleus into two parts, exchange one half of its nucleus for half the nucleus of the other paramoecium, via the mouth, and this is followed after various stages of nuclear change by each paramoecium splitting into two. There is no apparent difference between the two animals; they have no male and female organs, but the nuclei evidently contain in each case a " male " and " female " portion—a certain unknown something which is necessary to rejuvenescence. We have here the progenitors of bisexuality; but autosexuality is still an essential factor in propagation.

Higher in the scale we find the hydra—a multicellular animal. Here again we find autosexuality. The hydra without the aid of another one can " bud off " a new living hydra; but we also find bisexuality, in that it forms in itself male and female cells which unite with one another to form a new hydra in true bisexual manner. It is both autosexual and bisexual and shows early traces of hermaphroditism.

Yet further, as evolution proceeds, we find the earthworm. Each worm contains the organs of both sexes—ovary and testes fully developed, and each worm needs fertilisation from another individual. They are true hermaphrodites, and bisexuality is fully established. *Inasmuch as the two worms are of the same sex—both being male as well as female—we may say that they are homosexual* ; they are attracted by worms of similar constitution. The same applies also to the paramoecium.*

As we ascend higher still in the scale we find that the male and female organs still persist in all animals, but that gradually one set of organs only is fully developed, the other remaining more or less rudimentary. Therefore, individual beings in their development have become differentiated into male and female very gradually. But right up to and including human beings we still find that every individual has some of the organs of both sexes present in varying degrees of development with even occasional true hermaphroditism. Thus in the male we have rudimentary breasts and nipples and a rudimentary uterus (*uterus masculinis*),

---

*Homosexual—Sexual attraction between members of the same sex, whether male or female.

and in the female we have the homologue of the penis in the clitoris and of the scrotum in the labia majora, and so on. Every individual is bisexual physically.

The main trend of psychic sexual development runs on similar lines, and we find this repeated in the life of all animals, even those of the highest development.

Autosexuality is exhibited in very early childhood. Many parents are much distressed to find their infants have a tendency towards masturbation, or show other forms of so-called sexual precocity and perversions. Moreover, infants show many other manifestations of sexuality, which fortunately for the peace of mind of their parents are not commonly recognised as possessing sexual significance. *However, this autosexuality is not abnormal.* It is a stage in the infantile development of sex, and will normally be replaced by other manifestations at a later date *if wrong methods of repression without sublimation do not take place.* But it will not all disappear from the unconscious mind; some autosexuality remains in the adult, but its form is changed.

Human beings are not alone in this retention of the autosexual instinct.* Dogs are well known to attempt onanism, stags perform the

* See "The Nature of Man."—*Metchnikoff.*

act against trees, cattle, horses and monkeys do the same; the female monkey, like the female human infant, obtains sexual gratification by rubbing its thighs together, as well as by handling itself.

At a later stage of life we find a further development. Schoolboys and schoolgirls have not much attraction for the opposite sex— indeed, they are often scornful of them, and look upon the other sex with a certain disdain. They, however, form very strong friendships with members of their own sex, and it is common knowledge that under adverse conditions of sublimation they touch, inspect and gratify one another's sexual desires by masturbation, etc. In other words, before the full development of the sexual organs they have strong *homosexual tendencies* which may or may not be conscious, and may or may not be repressed and sublimated according to circumstances. Again we see a homosexual tendency in dogs, and other animals. (By homosexual tendencies is meant sexual attraction towards members of the *same* sex whether occurring in males or females. Heterosexual tendencies are those which are directed to members of the opposite sex). Here also there is no abrupt change from homo- to heterosexuality. Even after puberty a good deal of the homosexual remains as a component of our complete sexual instinct, but under normal circumstances it is either repressed or sublimated.

Finally then, at puberty we reach the normal attraction for members of the opposite sex (heterosexuality). But the other forms of sexuality still remain, although unconscious, and their energy is turned to other purposes, or partially so.

We might thus put down the sexuality of an infant as:

Autosexuality 100%

of a child of twelve years of age:

Autosexuality 40%
Homosexuality 50%
Heterosexuality 10%

of a *normal* individual at puberty:

Autosexuality 20%
Homosexuality 30%
Heterosexuality 50%

Any or all of these components may be:

(1) Repressed and then sublimated.
(2) Repressed without adequate sublimation, (causing neuroses, bad habits, etc).
(3) Not repressed, but expressed.
(4) Displaced.

These three forms of sexuality may be termed the *primary sexual aims, i.e.,* the individual aims at discharging his erotic energy through one of these channels. We are for the moment ignoring the fact that sublimation and displacement into other channels may take place.

Now if at any period of the child's life the normal psychic sexual development is interfered with or arrested the more primitive flow of energy along autosexual or homosexual lines may persist in the adult. Or should resistances which occur in adult life dam back the normal flow of energy through the heterosexual channel it may find its outlet through either of the more primitive channels. The two factors which appear to decide relative proportion of these forms of sexuality in the individual are:

(1) Heredity: constitutional tendency.
(2) Early environment.

Of these, heredity plays the smaller part. Early environment is nearly everything.

Thus far we have traced the development of the sexual aim; but we have by no means solved here the question of how the *sexual impulse* (or desire) as we know it is constituted; and again we must try to follow up some of the motives of the more primitive types of life.

In considering the impulses which go to make sexuality we shall see how some of these also serve the instinct of self-preservation and only secondarily acquire a sexual import.

One of the most important of the factors in the self-preservation of the primitive animal is *pain*. Pain is a warning to the animal that all is not well with it. Pain comes from wounds, from aggression of other animals ; it is an early warning of the finality of individual life. Hence the avoidance of pain and of such situations as lead to pain is in itself an act of self-preservation. But in the struggle for life which brings about the survival of the fittest mere avoidance of pain is not enough. Perhaps there is food for but one mouth ; there are two hungry mouths waiting. It is no longer a question of avoiding pain, but of aggression and of giving pain. The stronger finds that the fear of imminent death which follows his aggression and consequent pain to the weaker causes fear, and that the weaker prefers to risk a distant death by starvation rather than the imminent death foreboded by the aggression. Hence *aggression* becomes a vital necessity in early life—to kill, or, failing that, to cause pain and its accompanying fear becomes an integral factor of life. To subdue others is a necessity which becomes an instinct.

Now as soon as we deal with bisexual animals we are met with two facts. *Firstly*, that the sexual moment or period of impulse of one animal does not necessarily correspond with that of the other, and since the first animal has already discovered that desires are attained by aggression the first animal becomes aggressive, and subdues the second animal forcibly, and probably painfully, while the sexual act is performed. Moreover, the second animal, at first associating such aggression and pain with fear of extermination will now associate it with a different impulse—that of sexuality.

Secondly, after the sexual act has been commenced by the aggressor without apparent danger to the life of the aggressed, there is a relief on the part of the latter. Moreover, in the higher animals the pleasure of the sexual act is induced in the aggressed, even though conscious desire was not present before. So that both the active and passive partners associate aggression and cruelty with the sexual act ; the one as a giver, the other as a recipient of pain. But since both animals have bisexual characteristics, as has already been shown, both may connect *psychically* the giving and receiving of pain with sexuality.

It is possible that this explanation is not correct in detail, and that the aggression and pleasure of cruelty in the primitive types is in itself the prime sexual pleasure ; but in either case, the fact remains that *the pleasure of giving and of receiving pain of some kind is one of the primitive sexual impulses,* which Freud has called " partial impulses," and which go towards making the complete adult sexual impulse.

This is illustrated in many ways. In its least repressed form we have open sadism (cruelty for its own sake) and masochism (the desire to feel pain). A patient of mine who was fairly normal in most respects related how as a boy he used to flog himself when he masturbated, in order to increase the pleasure. In many of the more passionate types of the southern races it is not uncommon to find that both men and women bite one another or otherwise inflict injury during the act of coitus, and they ascribe added pleasure to the act thereby. Cruelty on the part of boys at school (bullying) is nearly always a sexual manifestation which, like homosexuality, should be only a passing phase, which is later repressed into the unconscious. The monks who denied themselves sexual intercourse, but found pleasure in flogging themselves or others, form an example of the way that sexual energy, when denied its normal course finds a more primitive outlet. A schoolmaster with repressed and unconscious homosexuality will often be noted for his flogging proclivities, and so forth. Children, more especially boys, are observed to have an instinct of cruelty ; for example they pull the wings off flies. The sport of the chase or of fishing serves to gratify the instinct in adults.

In connection with this subject of pain we now come to an important law. *EVERY FORM OF PSYCHIC ENERGY CAN MANIFEST ITSELF IN TWO WAYS, OF WHICH ONE IS DIAMETRICALLY OPPOSED TO THE OTHER.*

Thus cruelty for cruelty's sake, though a normal sexual impulse is recognised by the community as detrimental under present conditions to the general welfare. Hence from our earliest infancy we are taught to view it with horror and to *repress* tendencies to cruelty. The opposite of cruelty is *pity* ; and pity is a form of the sublimation* of cruelty. Analysis shows that the more an individual displays pity the more his unconscious mind contains of *repressed* cruelty.

As cruelty may be either towards another or towards oneself (in autosexual types), so pity, its sublimation, may be either towards others, or in autosexual types towards oneself (self pity). The person who is always desiring pity or sympathy is always one in whom environment and force of circumstance have prevented a flow of sexual energy into hetero-

---

*Pity and other "opposite manifestations" are not true sublimations. The reason of this will be found in a later chapter. They are better termed "negative to" their opposite.

sexual (or homosexual) channels, and the energy then endeavours to escape through autosexual channels. Thus there is no virtue in pity: it is not a question of the will, but purely of the emotions and is nothing else than one of the components of erotic desire.

Very much more might be said on this subject of cruelty and pity, but it is my object here to confine myself to just sufficient to indicate the general bearing on the subject. Much more research will be required before the whole matter in some of its complicated aspects is quite clear.

We now have to pass on to consider shortly other impulses which go to form the complex desire of sexuality. Some of the chief ones are as follows :

(1). *The desire to touch—contact—*is one of the most important of our erotic impulses. Not only is contact of the genital organs one of the main erotic desires but also contact of various parts of the body. It is obvious in the case of many of our progenitors that this played a very important part in leading up to the final sexual act. Thus if we consider the earliest forms of life that have no intellectual or reasoning power, and also have no actual reproductive organs, it is obvious that they cannot reason and say, " I must get near and touch the other individual in order to satisfy my sexuality !" The impulse to get near and touch the other individual must *in itself* be a predominant impulse. Contact of body itself must constitute the main impulse of a sexual nature in many instances. Thus in the paramoecium ; two of these animals come ventrally together and afterwards exchange nuclei through their mouths. One can hardly imagine that this primitive unicellular animal first desires to exchange a nucleus and then reasons that it must get close to and lie alongside the other one in order to do so. Its obvious impulse is first to come into contact with the whole of the under surface of another individual, and the sexual act is merely consummated by the actual discharge of the nuclei. Chemio-taxis may be the original motive power behind their drawing together, but whatever it be it is obvious that this is the first and essential part of the sexual operation.

As we follow the scale of evolution we see a similar condition of affairs, though in a modified degree. The earthworm is first attracted to lie alongside its mate, which it does for a considerable period before a " sexual act " take place. Again, many animals that have prolonged contact with one another's bodies *never have actual contact of the reproductive organs ;*

this applies especially to those in which the genital organs are not of an external nature, but in both sexes open merely into a vestibule (the cloaca) in common with the excretory organs. Thus the male frog clasps the female frog's body for hours on end; but no connection of male with reproductive female organs follows.

One can see the same in human beings. Contact of hands, lips (kissing), fondling of breasts, hair, face or skin nearly always precedes and leads up to the final sexual act. Indeed, without some such preliminary work many people find it difficult to have a sexual act at all—the repression of early environment being too great. Thus bodily contact in varying degrees is one of the pleasures and essential sexual components of the act of propagation.

We must now consider some of the details of this contact of body, as they play an important part in the sexual development of the human being. One knows that engaged persons delight to hold hands, to kiss ardently, to take one another's arms in walking, to stroke the hair, etc.; all these are sexual acts, and tend towards making the sexual consummation, although repression prevents the latter taking place or even entering into the conscious mind in many instances. Sometimes we find women who delight in taking another woman's hands or in caressing her or in kissing her. In this instance we may always know that there is a good deal of homosexuality present in the unconscious : again, it is a sexual act. Repressed homosexuality and autosexuality is much greater in women than in men on the whole, as they are brought up with much more repression and remain partially fixed in an infantile condition of sexuality, which will be discussed in the next chapter.

Erogenous Zones. Having shown that the sense of touch of the body in general has a very large sexual significance, Freud has designated certain parts of the body which have a special sexual significance erogenous zones. It is true that the activities of these erogenous zones are not confined to the sense of touch alone, but that seeing, smelling, hearing, etc., all have their part in the sexual activity of these zones. Nevertheless, the present place seems suitable for discussing them briefly.

The chief erogenous zones are as follows : the anus, the neck of the bladder, the mouth, breasts, eyes, hands, hair, feet, and the inner parts of the thighs.

The Anus.—Developmentally the anus and genital organs are lined with the same continuous mucous membrane. In the frog, bird and other primitive types they open into a common vestibule—the cloaca. They are very closely connected not only developmentally but functionally. Both the penis and anus are excretory, and the nerve supply of the sphincter and other muscles of both is of like origin. Thus we can see that in the primitive mind there is likely to be a very close connection between the anus and genital organs, and this is actually the case. In children this connection is strongly developed. They are taught to repress references connected with both organs, and they look upon them as similar in many ways. Moreover, following the developmental innervation of both there is a similar pleasure to be obtained with both, and just as one gets *referred pain* in the area of certain nerve supplies so one gets *referred pleasure*. Children often gain a considerable amount of pleasure from constipation, the hard fæces extending the anal sphincter in passing causing this, and the pleasure is sometimes referred to the genital organs. I have a patient at the time of writing who was always constipated as a child, and whose mother was in the habit of passing a soaped finger into the child's rectum in order that she might be induced to defæcate. The patient gained very considerable pleasure from this act of her mother, and often had a desire to kiss her mother during the process. In hysterical patients we often find an actual sexual sensation developed in connection with the mucous membrane of the anus. In children (and adults) enhanced pleasure is experienced by pressure on the anus during masturbation, and the same is true of many married persons during normal coitus. Some persons without any apparent cause have a habit of scratching or rubbing the neighbourhood of the anus. Psychoanalysis has shown that this anal sexuality exists in a repressed form in everybody. Its degree, of course, varies enormously ; in some persons it is completely repressed and unconscious : in other persons (adults) it assumes the form of a perversion, and they delight to have actual sexual connection *per anum.* Various intermediate forms exist : the patient I referred to above delights in becoming constipated and in removing her fæces with her own finger, now that she has grown up and her mother's ministrations are no longer possible.

The main point is that anal eroticism is a normal sexual impulse in infancy, but that in the normal individual it becomes repressed and sublimated. The anus in a perverted male often represents by association and development the vagina : it is a further example of his psychic bisexuality.

The Mouth.—The mouth has in some senses even more sexual import than the anus. We have seen that its use in the most primitive of types, *i.e.*, in the paramoecium, is not only nutritional, but that the actual sexual act takes place by an exchange of nuclei through the mouth. Higher in the scale, the hydra has but one opening into the exterior, which answers the purpose of both mouth and anus. Dogs and other animals often lick their own and other animals' genital organs. When we come to human beings association gives it a still greater significance as an organ of sexual impulse. The lips of the vaginal orifice (*labia*) have by association of ideas a strong similarity to those of the mouth ; the fact that they have been named the *labia* is evidence of the psychic connection. The tongue often has a similar association with the penis. One of the commonest of all adult perversions is that involving either the tongue or lips of one individual with the genital organs of the other. In hysterias and in dreams we find (by psycho-analysis) that there is a frequent displacement from below upwards on the body, *i.e.*, that parts of the upper portion of the body—mouth, teeth, head, breasts, etc.—become symbolic of the lower (genital) organs, which are repressed. Thus all forms of kissing are sexual impulses ; everyone knows how strongly sexual this impulse is between persons of the opposite sex, but even with persons of the same sex this touching of the lips is strongly sexual, though the sexuality is repressed into the unconscious and it is often merely homosexually symbolic of the touching of the reproductive organs. Not only is touch of sexual significance in the function of the mouth, but so also is sight. The desire to look at a woman's lips, the novelists' description of them as " tempting lips," " full lips," " delicate lips," etc., are all merely descriptions of their sexual attraction. The woman who rouges her lips shows an exhibition complex.* She calls attention to the lips of her mouth instead of to the labia majora— *the sexual idea is repressed into the unconscious, the sexual impulse still finding a primitive and symbolic outlet.* Thumb sucking in a child is a masturbation substitute in which both lips and hand have sexual significance ; nail biting is a variant of this.

Similar symbolic significances are by displacement attached to the eyes and the hair, etc.

The Breasts, of course, have an actual sexual significance as well as a nutritive one, and there are few lovers who have not on many occasions

* Complex.   A repressed group or constellation of ideas,

found touching and fondling the breasts with the hands of considerable erotic significance previous to the final act of coitus.

The Hands have acquired a true sexual significance with an altogether bisexual value. From touching the breasts, genitals, etc., to stroking the hair, skin, etc., this significance is very apparent (*cf.* the clasping of the female by the male forelimbs in lower animals). Again, in dreams we find the hands frequently symbolic of actual reproductive organs and with reproductive functions. The touch of the skin anywhere affords one of the outlets for the sexual impulses (the pain and pleasure impulse of masochism and sadism, and their reverse).

(2). *The desire to look at (inspection) and its counterpart, the desire to be looked at (exhibition).*

Here again we have the aggressive or active and the aggressed or passive desire present in both sexes just as we have in the desire for cruelty, and for similar reasons, *i.e.*, that all individuals are bisexual. This again, in autosexual types, becomes a desire to look at oneself.

The desire to look probably comes from the necessity to look. In those animals where senses of smell, hearing, and so forth are not sufficient to distinguish the sex of another individual, it becomes a necessity to examine the reproductive organs of the other individual in order to see whether a suitable aim for the discharge of erotic energy is present. In the passive case (the female) when an impulse towards desiring aggression is present, there the converse is true, *i.e.*, the desire to exhibit the reproductive organs, so that the aggressor should recognise his possibilities. In time this desire to look and be looked at becomes extended, and other parts of the body are included as well as the genital organs. Thus in the peacock and many other animals we see the desire extended to the *tail* feathers ; *i.e.*, the parts in the neighbourhood of the reproductive organs acquire a suggestive significance. Women's evening dress is an unconscious display of the same type.

It is true that in the example of the peacock it is the male which exhibits himself, and in other types it is the female. But it must be remembered that *all* individuals are bisexual, and have both the desire to exhibit and to inspect. Which of these desires is in the ascendant in any particular type of male or female depends upon its environment and its racial and individual evolution and on the course which " natural selection " has been compelled to take.

This exhibition tendency is seen in very young children. It is well known that the infant of two or three years old loves to be undressed and to strut about before an admiring circle of friends. "Come and see me bathed" is a frequent request made by a child to a visitor of whom he or she is particularly fond. In this case we have the passive form of exhibitionism. In the active form children delight to peep through keyholes to see other individuals without their clothes, etc., etc. The desire to exhibit their genital organs is more strong in females than in males in whom the desire to look is stronger as a rule. Moreover, by association the desire is transferred to other "erotic zones," *i.e.*, the desire to look at the skin, the breasts, the mouth, the anus, the hair, the eyes and general shape. Indeed, we can see from this that the idea of beauty in human beings is a purely arbitrary one, based on the conscious conception of sex. In the South Sea Islands the greatest beauty may consist in a flat nose ; in Rome of an aquiline nose ; in other countries, of some other type of nose.

Indeed, artists who make a speciality of figure painting are *displacing* a strong exhibition tendency, while those who paint other pictures of Nature may be said to be sublimating their tendency.

By sublimation we mean changing the energy of sexual desire into activities which have no sexual meaning.

By displacement we mean changing the energy into another form of sexuality which though disguised is yet fully sexual.

Now the community has decreed for various reasons (some of which are good and others bad) that this desire to look and to be looked at is unwholesome : therefore we are taught to repress it, with two results.

Firstly, it may be changed to its opposite —*shame* and *modesty* (*cf.* cruelty—pity). And since women have the innate desire to exhibit more strongly developed and from infancy are more strongly taught to repress all things pertaining to sex, so in women are shame and modesty more highly developed.

' As in the case of pity there is no virtue in " modesty " ; it is one of those characteristics purely dependent on the early environment of the individual, and the more marked it is the stronger is the *unconscious* impulse of exhibitionism in that individual. Indeed, it is well known to many (quite apart from the facts elicited by psycho-analysis) that the child with the greatest exhibition tendencies grows up the most modest and has the most shame ; and moreover, that under suitable circumstances (hysterias, etc.) after reaching puberty the most modest person may become the most shameless exhibitionist.

Secondly, this exhibition tendency, instead of sublimating itself as its antithesis, may *project* itself, *i.e.*, it may be displaced from the actual person on to things belonging to or surrounding the person. The best example of this is seen again in dress, and once again in women's dress more often than in men's. To exhibit oneself in fine clothing (and on the part of the other sex, to admire the one in fine clothing) is merely a displacement of the sexual impulse of exhibitionism. While in cases where there is a good deal of repression of *normal* sexuality, and hence a return to the *infantile* autosexuality, we have the desire to look at oneself and examine one's own reproductive organs or body, transformed into a desire to wear beautiful underclothing,* and so forth—shame preventing the actual primitive impulse from being gratified. These methods are all very low types of substitution, however, and as we shall see at a later period, by no means useful *now* to the community ; and no doubt evolution, which is gradually tending towards the intellectual rather than the physical will bring forward non-differentiation of men and women in clothing, hairdressing, and so forth. At present about nine-tenth of our shops, adver-

---

*Narcisistic and parental complexes also play their part in this partioular oaoc.

tisements and pleasures are engaged upon accentuating this form of sexual exhibitionism in one way or another. The early Puritans and Quakers evidently partly realised these points, as is shown by their manner of dress and writings.

From the eye we pass on to the other organs —those of hearing and smelling in connection with sex. Of hearing we need say little ; it plays its part in the love-making of birds especially, but is also found in other animals. The song of the bird in the breeding season is not far removed from the human lover's voice, praising the visual charms of the loved one, or giving vent to songs which bring to the imagination the pleasures of sex in their disguised and sublimated forms.

Smelling also plays its part. In many animals the distinctive smell of the male and female organs is of great importance in distinguishing sex, and it cannot be denied that it gradually assumes a sexual pleasure and impulse of its own : moreover, the anus being situated close to the reproductive organs the sense of smell of the one is always associated with the sense of smell of the other. Anyone who has watched two dogs or a dog and a bitch smelling the genital and excretory organs of the other and wagging their tails in evident pleasure will realise this. It will similarly be realised why dogs apparently smell one another's excrement with pleasure, and why when they discover the spot where another dog has micturated they through association of ideas do the same at the same place.

Now in children there is also a considerable liking for the smell of excrement and in adults it sometimes persists (again depending on environment and amount of repression). The community of humans, however, has placed its ban upon the open enjoyment of this form of erotic impulse, and its opposite becomes its sublimation—disgust and loathing of excrement and its accompanying smell, and also by association, of any smell suggestive of it, *e.g.*, rotten eggs, onions, garlic, etc. And the greater the normal inclination of the individual towards this pleasure of sexual smell the greater does his loathing become on account of its repression.

We deduce then that sexual impulses are many and varied, and that the final act of coitus is but one of many. Moreover, that any of these sexual impulses may have auto-sexual, homosexual or heterosexual aims according to various circumstances which will be discussed in the next chapter.

SUMMARY

1. *A large amount of psychic energy originally devoted to self-preservation has been diverted towards self-propagation. Modern sexuality, therefore, is greater than is necessary or desirable, and much energy might be sublimated along intellectual or physical paths.*

2. *All individuals are bisexual both physically and psychically.*

3. *Sexual aims are of three kinds—the autosexual, the homosexual, the heterosexual. Each is normal at successive stages of life.*

4. *The sexual impulse is made up of many partial impulses, and is not in itself merely the impulse towards a definite act of coitus with one of the opposite sex.*

5. *Early teaching and environment cause us to repress both sexual aims and sexual impulses whether normal or abnormal, into the unconscious. Adult sexuality depends on the type and amount of such repression and on the type and amount of compensatory sublimation obtained.*

CHAPTER IV

The Fate of Erotic Impulses and Erotic Aims

In the last chapter we discussed the question of psycho-sexual energy, aims and impulses, and we regarded the latter as being a kind of connecting link between the erotic energy and the erotic aims. We have now to consider what happens normally to these impulses and aims and also what may abnormally take place.

In actual life three things which we have illustrated in the last chapter may happen; namely, in the first place, the primitive instincts may be manifested with but little repression; in the second place, they may be repressed and shown in a disguised form; in the third place, they may be repressed and sublimated. For example: as regards the exhibition tendency, it may proceed through life as a desire either to exhibit or to look at the reproductive organs and erogenous zones, according to the predominant factor in the bisexual tendency of the individual; it may displace itself by hiding the desire to be looked at in so far as the reproductive organs are concerned and show itself in the desire to

63

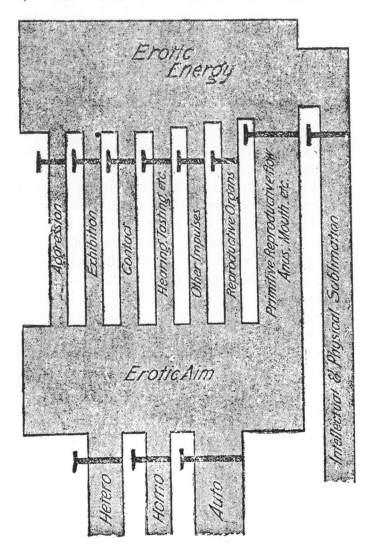

be looked at (or to look at) in relation to clothing or to other parts of the body. Thirdly, it may be sublimated into intellectual or physical pursuits. This applies not only to the exhibition tendency just quoted, but to all the other forms of erotic impulses previously enumerated and shown in the accompanying diagram.

In this diagram the primitive energy is shown as contained in a tank labelled " erotic energy," with various pipes leading from it. These pipes represent the outlets for the following infantile tendencies (primitive impulses), namely—aggression, exhibition, contact, impulses of the reproductive organs, and impulses connected with other parts of the body (anus, mouth, etc.) ; an overflow pipe is also shown, which conducts the impulses of intellectual and physical sublimation. As I have previously explained, the overflow pipe will not carry the whole, but a great part of the energy, and it will be observed that in the figure that it does not drain the tank and is not placed quite at the bottom thereof : in other words, however much we sublimate our energy there is always some left over which must flow through primitive channels or remain in the tank, and this amount depends on the efficiency of the individual, which in its turn depends largely on early environment. Now all these erotic impulses are further shewn in the figure to flow into a second tank, which has been labelled "erotic aims"; we have demonstrated already these aims to be three in number—namely, autosexual, homosexual and heterosexual. Three large pipes are placed beneath this tank and represent the outlets for these three " aims."

Let us suppose now that each pipe may be opened or closed by means of a tap. It will at once be seen what a great variety of results may occur by means of closing or opening some of these taps either in whole or in part, and at the same time keeping others closed.

If we regard this tank of erotic energy with its various pipes from the point of view of what may happen in childhood, we see that in infancy it is possible to turn off (by parental education and general environment) several of the taps, and so force the flow of energy through only one or two of the pipes : for instance, the taps in the pipes labelled exhibitionism and aggression may be fully opened and all others closed ; in which case we produce a shameless child (exhibitionism) who is cruel and a bully (aggression), or one who, by sublimation, is very modest and prudish (the negative of exhibitionism), and timorous and full of pity (the negative of aggression). The same principle, of course, applies to any of the other impulses. If, however, we reach puberty before the actual repression occurs (*i.e.*, before the taps are turned off) we have a different series of events, but with a similar ultimate result. For instance, if on account of circumstances the normal heterosexual outlet is blocked, the pent-up force will then partly be damned back, and will be obliged to flow through one of the subsidiary pipes, *i.e.*, either that of homosexuality, autosexuality, or the overflow pipe of sublimation. If it be also turned off rather higher up in, say, all the outlets belonging to the reproductive organs, it will have to choose between aggression and its variations, exhibition and its variations and so forth. As an example, suppose a woman to be brought up to the age of puberty in an apparently normal manner. Owing to training and environment hetero-sexual and autosexual taps are turned off. This leaves only a flow through homosexuality. Owing to further circumstances (partially dating back to infantile years) *all* impulses for the reproductive outlets are then closed. We have left aggression (and its reverse), exhibitionism (and its reverse), as *impulses*, and homosexuality as the *aim*. The characteristics of that person will then be as follows : cruelty or extreme pity (repressed aggression) towards *members of the same sex ;* delight in extravagant clothing (or extreme simplicity and puritanical views on the same).   These characteristics represent the erotic impulses.   As for the erotic aim (homosexual) she will avoid men, seek the company of women, delight in women's friendships of an exaggerated nature in which profuse kissing, holding of hands, etc., takes place, according to the outlets which have their taps most fully open, but since the taps for the reproductive organ impulses are closed, she will not be conscious of any homosexual desire in connection with these organs.

Or again, take a boy in whom all the taps in the " impulse " pipes are closed except those of anal-eroticism and the reproductive organs, and also the taps in the " aim " pipes of hetero-sexual and homosexual aims. He will be autosexual, and the autosexuality will be satisfied with constipation (anal-erotic) and later (for reasons to be explained in a future place) with the desire to collect—stamps, butterflies, etc., (this represents the anal-erotic impulse), and he will be a masturbator (the reproductive organ impulse with an autosexual aim).   At a later date he may be very precise, careful and miserly (anal-erotic impulse).

Of course, we should rarely get a simple case in which some of the taps were completely turned off and others fully open. These simple illustrations will be complicated by the fact that there are many subsidiary impulses not shown in the diagram, and that most of the taps would at least be partially open in varying degrees. In all the above cases we have assumed that the pipe labelled sublimation is partly closed. Had this not been the case we might for instance have our exhibitionist sublimating his desires and becoming a decorative painter, or a scientist whose desire to look was now turned into research work in which he used a microscope, etc. Thus is future character formed by early environment.

From the points already mentioned in this chapter three terms arise which are in common use : repression, perversion and regression.

Repression.—By repression we mean that infantile or primitive instincts, impulses and aims have been forced completely into the unconscious mind, or have, by environment and education been prevented from becoming conscious at all. The complexes and ideas connected with these primitive impulses are dissociated from the conscious mind.

Perversion.—In the case of perversions we deal with a condition in which adequate repression does not take place, and infantile tendency remains throughout youth and puberty. Thus, if the infantile tendency and environment have been towards homosexual aims the adult remains an acknowledged homosexual, or if the infantile tendency is largely aggressive the adult remains brutal in sexual matters; if the male tendency is in the ascendant his idea is to capture the female by force, or if the female tendency, it is to be captured by force, and so forth. (*Cf.* masochism or sadism). The term perversion merely means that some infantile or primitive erotic aim remains active and unchanged at or after puberty.

Regression.—Finally, regression means that the individual, owing to later environment, is forced to abandon normal erotic aims and impulses, and, having the path for sublimation blocked, is obliged to allow the dammed back energy to flow once more through infantile channels; thus, if normal heterosexual channels are blocked we may find autosexuality, with accompanying masturbation or we may find all actual reproductive outlets closed and nothing left open except either exhibition or aggression ; in which case murderers and lunatics may be the result. But if the tap of the pipe of sublimation be left open a large portion of this excess erotic energy may flow over and deleterious results may thus be entirely avoided.

To summarise : repression means that the infantile erotic desires are pushed into the unconscious mind and kept there, If the repression ceases, or has never taken place, a perversion results—a perversion being any infantile erotic aim or impulse which persists after the infantile stage has been passed. Regression is a lapse into the infantile tendency and either leads to a perversion or to a sexual repression. Strictly speaking, all artificial differentiation of sex, such as women's clothing, and so forth, is a perversion of sex ; but we have grown used to looking upon it as normal in spite of the fact that it is in reality merely an infantile exhibit on-ism which is displaced. This leads us to consider the terms displacement and sublimation more fully.

Displacement implies that the energy of an erotic impulse has been forced from its obvious path, which is sexual, into another path which is still sexual in its aim but is so disguised that the individual does not recognise it in its true form. It is a kind of self-deception, and still retains its strong erotic nature.

Sublimation is more than a displacement ; in it the energy of an erotic impulse is turned into a channel which is no longer sexual but is either purely intellectual or physical ; *emotion, however, must be attached to it still—i.e.,* pleasure or excitement must be obtained from the new work. Thus, if exhibitionism be turned into attractive clothing we have a displacement ; if the energy be turned into religion, music, scientific pursuits or hockey we have a sublimation. Now more than one form of displacement can occur. We may either have a displacement along the ordinary lines of everyday life, such as have already been exemplified, or we may have another sort of displacement depending upon the amount of resistance present and the particular type of infantile perversion attempting to come to the surface— an abnormal type — when we may have fetishism, or one of the diseases known as the psycho-neuroses.

Fetishism is displacement in which our erotic impulse is concentrated upon an object which in itself has no erotic significance but is merely symbolic of the true sexual aim. Thus a woman may treasure a rose worn by her lover, or a man place great value on a glove, handkerchief, or lock of hair. This is occasionally carried to excess in pathological conditions, and we may find that an individual's sole erotic aim consists in stroking hair or worshipping some article of clothing. The original impulse, instead of carrying him to its normal aim, has stopped halfway, and in itself become an aim. In the case of a psychoneurosis, however, a totally different state of affairs occurs. The infantile impulse which is trying to gain consciousness is strongly resisted by the censor of the conscious mind, (of which censor we shall speak in the next chapter), and instead of reaching consciousness in its infantile form it expends its energy in either a physical or a mental disability, which goes by the name of a psycho-nuerosis, or " functional " disease, the mechanism of which, as being of considerable importance, will have two future chapters to itself.

There is a third way in which these infantile erotic wishes and their repressed conflicts with the conscious mind find outlet, and that is in dreams.

. It is well at this point to make it quite clear that the repressed material found in psychoanalysis is by no means chiefly of a grossly sexual nature. All kinds of unpleasant conflicts are repressed. Conflicts of duty as opposed to pleasure or expediency—every kind of unpleasant idea which we try to avoid and repress is present. But underlying all the psychoneuroses we find various forms of misplaced psychic energy, belonging to some erotic infantile impulse or aim dammed back, and it is for this reason that these aims and impulses must be specially dwelt upon. They are those which normally we refuse to consider as part of our psychic individuality.

SUMMARY OF CHAPTER IV

1. *The main characteristics of an individual depend largely on which of his erotic impulses are encouraged and which repressed during infancy, and upon the amount of sublimation attained.*

2. *If circumstances arise at puberty or after, which are inimical to the normal flow of erotic energy, the energy will tend to seek an outlet through the channels which were most widely open in infancy—i.e., regression takes place.*

3. *Repression is necessary for the normal existence of the individual, but suitable sublimation contemporaneously is of the utmost importance.*

4. *Where adequate sublimation has not been attained, there is a tendency to use displacement, especially in females under present methods of education and environment. Displacement is waste of psychic energy and is often harmful to the community.*

CHAPTER V

PARENTAL COMPLEXES*

THE most important factor in the formation of the character of any individual is the influence of the parents. This is a self-evident fact; but what, unfortunately, is not so evident is that the influence which acts most powerfully on the child's existence is not the conscious, directive and educational influence but the unconscious, seemingly unimportant details of behaviour and speech, which so many parents would believe to be of little or no effect in the formation of the young child's character. This belief is shown by analysis to be absolutely wrong. *Unconsidered and apparently trivial details in the behaviour of the parents during the first five years of the child's life make a far greater impression on its mind and have far more weight in the formation of its character than any other factors occurring later.*

Before going into the details of this it is necessary to discuss shortly the problem of incest, for one of the mistakes that is most

*A complex is a constellation or group of ideas which is repressed into the unconscious or which has never been conscious.

commonly made is that since Christianity has
drawn up the table of affinity forbidding marriage between near relatives therefore no sexual
attraction between such normally exists. This
assumption is very wide of the mark, and in the
case of the small child in the first year or so of
its life it is in every instance the reverse of true.
Children are primitive creatures ; their unconscious feelings have very little repression ;
their instincts are the primitive instincts of their
fore-fathers, and they remain primitive until
education and environment—however elementary the nature of these—shall have repressed
and moulded them. It will be remembered
that the Incas of Peru and certain ruling castes of
Egypt were obliged to marry their own sisters,
and that children were born to them : nor was
this looked upon as an incestuous practice by
these peoples. Such marriages still take place
amongst certain primitive tribes. Among animals, even those of the highest types such as the
dog, no incest barrier exists : not only do
brothers and sisters of the dog family have
sexual relationship but mothers and sons, especially if the mother be young at the time the son
is born. Thus the question of affinity is chiefly
one of religion and early training and not of the
natural instincts of the unconscious.

Actual analysis shows that in practically

every normal human being the first love of a
son is for his mother, and of a daughter for her
father, and that this love is of a sexual nature,
although of course this does not necessarily mean
sexual as applied to the reproductive organs
but that the infantile, erotic impulses of touch,
sight, aggression, or whatever they may be, are
attracted by the parent of the opposite sex, and
that a certain erotic bond which we term
" *fixation* " is formed between the child and that
parent. This fixation varies in strength according to circumstances, and according to its
strength is formed the subsequent love type
of that particular child. It is not necessarily
upon the parent that the fixation is formed :
if the parent dies, or lives apart during the
child's infancy the fixation would be directed
towards whoever may take that parent's place—
the parent's substitute. The two complexes
that are thus formed are respectively termed
the *Œdipus Complex*, *i.e.*, the love of the son for
the mother, and the *Electra Complex*, *i.e.*, the
love of the daughter for her father, or more
commonly they are both included under the term
Œdipus Complex, after the play by Sophocles,
in which Œdipus unknowingly married his
mother. Freud terms these the nuclear complexes.

In the normal individual this fixation serves

its purpose, is gradually repressed, and the
energy behind it is then transferred to other
love objects ; and it will be found that if the
fixation has been fairly strong in childhood the
type of man that the adult woman marries
corresponds in a high degree to the father upon
whom there was this early fixation, and *vice
versa* in the case of the son and his mother.
This is borne out in a striking manner by
records of cases in which the daughter of a
drunkard will marry a drunkard, the daughter
of an old man a man much older than herself,
or a daughter who has much admired some
mental attribute in her father will marry a man
who has this attribute very strongly defined ;
and the same applies to the choice by a man of
his wife.   Although of course in both instances
the resemblance is not very marked to the out-
sider it will nearly always be found by
analysis.   There is one exception to this rule,
and that is where a fixation has been so strong
and so near the surface that marriage with a love
type strikingly like the parent in any respect
would bring the incestuous impulses of the child
towards the parent too near the surface.   Here
if marriage takes place we may find the chosen
one to possess attributes, especially those of a
physical kind, of exactly the opposite to those
of the parent.   The daughter of an extremely

well-built father would for instance marry a small, thin man, upon exactly the same principle which we have discussed in an earlier chapter— that the exact opposite often disguises a strong primitive instinct of an infantile character and prevents it from becoming conscious. (*Cf.*, aggression and pity ; exhibitionism and modesty, etc.)

In psycho-analysis this Œdipus complex is nearly always found to be strongly marked and of the utmost importance, for it often lies at the root of the whole of a patient's troubles. Any superabundance of affection on the part of the parent will cause the fixation to be too strong for normal repression or for transference to take place. Thus we often find that the " only " child who is much spoiled and petted becomes the subject of a psychoneurosis based on these complexes. It is a common practice for mothers to fondle their children, to hold them tightly, to kiss them affectionately, and to allow them, for instance, to come into their beds in the early morning ; and by all these actions they are naturally arousing the primitive sexual impulses in the unconscious of the infant. These impulses, as has been previously explained, have nothing to do in the early stages with the reproductive organs, but merely act upon all the other manifold erotic zones that we have already discussed. Later they may unconsciously affect the reproductive organs also. In the case of a boy a very strong fixation upon the mother may now be formed ; in the case of a girl, upon whom the mother does not as a rule shower quite so much exuberant affection, a weaker homosexual affection may be formed. The father who idolises his infant daughter may in the same way produce a fixation, perhaps even before the infant can walk and talk.

Now suppose that this exuberant affection is repressed after the first three or four years of the child's life, and becomes apparently more normal when the age of the child is five or six ; let us see what may result. Firstly, the child may grow up with an exaggerated notion of its duty towards the parent of the opposite sex ; secondly, it may never discover a mate whose perfections come up to the perfection of the parent ; thirdly, if it should discover such a mate, its unconscious fixation upon the parent and the resemblance of the mate to that parent will often create a kind of unconscious identification of the mate with the parent ; then the actual conscious sexual intercourse with the mate becomes a form of incest, with the result that we get a case of sexual impotence in the man, or of sexual anæsthesia* in the woman,

* Sexual impotence and sexual anæsthesia have many other infantile causes besides the one explained, most of them, however, lend themselves to analysis.

and since the spoiling of the daughter by her father is by no means an uncommon occurrence, so we find sexual anæsthesia and sexual disgust on the part of a wife towards her husband a fairly common occurrence, which can only be rectified by analysis of this Œdipus complex ; and even then, if the fixation is very strong we may find the analysis a long and difficult one. Another result which may follow is that a strong fixation upon the parent of the opposite sex prevents any transference of erotic energy to other members of the opposite sex : and if the erotic impulses of this individual be very strong we find them turned off into the easier channels of homosexuality, where they become fixed.

This homosexuality may be conscious and practised and carried on into adult life : or it may be repressed and either sublimated, as in the case of strong friendships with members of the same sex, or it may be permitted to retain its primitive infantile erotic impulses, quite apart from the reproductive organs, and result in those cases which we see of women who delight to hold hands, to kiss one another rather passionately, to visit one another's bedrooms and inspect clothing, and to give evidence of this sexuality in a thousand and one other displaced forms. This sort of thing is more noticeable in women than men, because strong parental fixation is more common in women, and their education and environment help to repress the normal sexual growth more than in the case of men. It is a common error to explain this by saying that women are more affectionate than men, whereas if men were to perform some of the acts which we have described, everyone would suspect them of being homosexual.

The true facts of the case are, then, that women have a much stronger leaning towards homosexuality than men, and this is owing to the early training and environment of women. But that this is so is not often recognised: and those who have a repressed or disguised complex will be the last to discover that complex in themselves. Thus many of the acts which we look upon as perfectly normal and natural should, in reality, be classed scientifically as perversions: while it will be seen that a vast number of harmful results may follow every abnormal fixation upon the parents: these are augmented when early fixation upon a brother or a sister, either of a homosexual or heterosexual nature, takes place. The fixation of a boy upon his mother may at her death, or upon some other occasion, be transferred to a sister who, in every respect is the nearest ideal to his mother, with the added advantage that she is younger: and the fixation may remain there permanently.

As a rule the stronger the fixation upon the parent of the opposite sex the stronger will become the jealousy, although repressed and unconscious, towards the parent of the same sex. The father becomes in the unconscious the rival of the son for the mother's affection. This is very commonly seen in an undisguised form in children : a boy will be pleased when his father is out in the evening and he can take his father's place at table. If his father is staying away it is usual for him to ask if he may sleep with his mother, and sometimes he will suggest playing at husband and wife and calling her by her christian name, or a thousand and one other playful and seemingly innocent childish remarks and actions of the boy trying to take his father's place will occur to almost anyone. Moreover, it is by no means uncommon to see from quite early infancy an antagonism between father and son—a desire on the part of the latter that the father should be out of the way : and should the father quarrel with his mother on the trivial matters of everyday life, as will occur in every household, the child will often fume and rage against his father as he either takes his mother's part or refrains from doing so with the greatest difficulty. Exactly the same may take place with the girl and her mother.

This repressed incest desire, with its accompanying jealousy and unconscious hatred breeds a sense of guilt, and this in turn will cause the child, or in later years the adult, to give on occasion exaggerated affection and deference to the parent of the same sex as a compensation for the exaggerated antagonism and hatred: and we have these two emotions very often alternating—antagonism one day or on one occasion, exaggerated affection and deference on the next, and these alternations of love and hate in a repressed form are found in a very large number of the compulsion neuroses, and in particular in that form of compulsion neurosis which has become known as *folie du doute.**

The dreams of patients bear out these statements.† It is by no means uncommon for the patient to dream of the death of the parent of his own sex ; that is to say, the wish fulfilment is present in the dream—not that the parent should actually die, but that he should be " out of the way." On the other hand, in nearly every neurotic patient we get at one time or another a series of unmistakeable sex dreams toward the parent of the opposite sex, as a

* In *folie du doute* we almost invariably find, as well as a strong parental fixation with alternating love and hate, three other unconscious infantile complexes strongly marked : anal-eroticism, exhibitionism and homosexuality.

† This part will not be completely understood until the next chapter, on " Dreams," has been read.

rule slightly disguised, but sometimes absolutely crude, much to the patient's disgust and indignation. Brill places on record thirty-eight dreams of sexual relation with the patient's mothers given to him by twenty-one patients with very little distortion. About half these dreamers reported the dreams before they had heard of the Œdipus complex, while the others told him after he had explained its mechanism and said that they had not told him before because they had thought them too terrible and revolting. He relates the same of nineteen women, who dreamed that they had sexual relations with their fathers. Much more often the dreams are slightly disguised, with the father or the mother masked. Thus one of Brill's female homosexual patients told him that the only dream in which a man had ever played a part was one in which she had dreamed that she had sexual intercourse with one of her governors : but in giving associations to the dream she said that she always referred to her father as " the governor," and, as is well-known by psychoanalysts, president, governor, priest, mayor, king etc., in dreams always refer to the father. More often, however, the personality of the parent or of the patient is quite recognisable : it is the sexual act itself which is disguised, and yet only faintly or by some very typical symbolism which the veriest beginner in analysis would recognise without having to ask for associations. Several excellent examples of these dreams are given in Brill's work on the *Theory and Practical Application of Psycho-Analysis.*

I have already referred to the fact that a fixation may often be turned from a parent to a brother or sister : and, moreover, that a fixation may tend to preserve the individual in the infantile homosexual state. These fixations may become very much more strongly established if brothers and sisters are allowed to occupy the same bedroom, or, worse still, sleep in the same bed. Again, there is no actual primitive incest barrier between brothers and sisters or between *brothers alone* or *sisters alone*, and homosexual and even heterosexual behaviour is quite common with children under such conditions. *It may often have very much more serious consequences if one girl sleeps with another girl or one boy with another boy than if in childhood members of the opposite sex are put to sleep together : the fixations underlying many unhappy psychoneuroses may then originate.*

Another variant of this parental complex is sometimes found, and that is a strong homosexual fixation on the parent of the same sex. It is brought about by circumstances similar to those which cause the Œdipus complex, and is especially marked where the parent of the opposite sex has died during the early infancy of the child, but this latter is by no means essential. It depends on the fact already mentioned that all individuals are bisexual, and that a woman in the unconscious as in the conscious, often plays the masculine role and the man a feminine one. Indeed, it must be recognised that the pleasure obtained by the female in actual sexual intercourse is created in the nerves of the clitoris, *i.e.*, in her *male reproductive organ* and hence is of the masculine type.

This brings us to mention shortly one of the reasons why neuroses and psychoneuroses are more common in women than in men and why they are more fixed in infantile sexuality as a rule. It is this—the female is in fact not very different from the male. As a child this is especially the case, but from a very early age she is surrounded by the artificial differentiation which civilisation has built up and she is forced into repressing her normal male instincts and assuming an exaggerated female pose. Skirts, exaggerated sex courtesys and various other follies are quickly thrust upon her with the result of very much repression and infantile fixation. She is made to become a more artificial product than the male in the early years when there should be no differentiation at all. Some observers have added the difficulty which a woman at puberty has of transferring her sexual centre of gratification in the organs of reproduction from the clitoris to the vagina. I do not agree with this, for having collected statistics from many sources besides that of my own patients I find that no such change takes place as a rule in *normal* women. The clitoris generally remains the essential seat of gratification, and in those cases where such a change is found it is, I believe, a return to an infantile erotic zone, in the neck of the bladder, the vagina, and the rectum—or perhaps more correctly it is a return to *cloacal eroticism.**

It will be seen then, that criminal parents may even in their neglect give their children a better chance than the most loving of parents give to their children. I have only quoted

*I used the term " cloacal eroticism " to designate the eroticism pertaining to all that region, except the penis and clitoris, supplied by the pudic branches of the sacral plexus ; *e.g.*, the anus, scrotum, labia majora, urethra, part of the vagina and perineum.   (Perineal eroticism is very common but has not, I think, been definitely mentioned by other authors hitherto.)

One must also include the skin on the inner part of the thigh under the same heading, since from its nerve supply, *e.g.*, genito-crural, it probably belongs to the same set of segments in the human body as the original cloaca.

The other nerve supply in this region is derived from the hypogastric plexus which supplies the vagina on the one hand and the prostate and region of the uterus masculinus on the other.

Developmentally, the vagina comes from the lower part of the Mullerian Ducts and is therefore of much older origin than the clitoris a few of the more striking actions of the parents which may have this undesirable influence, but 't must be remembered that a very large number of other seemingly unnoticed acts and habits of the parents are taking their share in determining the strength of the infantile parental fixation. I will now give two or three examples of actual cases in order to illustrate the mechanism of what we have been discussing.

Case 1.—A patient, a man whose father was austere and very strict, and whose mother was more than usually affectionate towards him in childhood gave a history in which all his youthful love episodes had been directed towards women considerably older than himself. At twenty-two he married a woman of thirty-eight, and found that he was almost, but not quite, sexually impotent towards her. She died, and shortly afterwards he again married a woman considerably older than himself. Analysis showed him that in both these cases he, without any doubt whatever, had seen the mother in the woman he

or penis ; it would therefore be much more in keeping with nature of evolution did we regard a displacement of sexual gratification from the clitoris to the vagina as a regression, rather than as the normal procedure.

This is borne out by the evidence which I have gathered from about 150 cases of apparently normal women, related to me by various doctors.

Of these, three were said to be completely anæsthetic, 14 were said to have pleasure chiefly referred to the vagina but without orgasm, in the remainder, without exception, the glans clitoris was the essential seat of sensation though about 60 of these cases also admitted very variable vaginal, perineal and anal sensations simultaneously.

married, and that in physical build and type of feature they were very much like his mother.

*Case 2.—A folie du doute** in a young man. A history of extreme affection for the mother with infantile jealousy towards the father was obtained very rapidly. Later, analysis brought to light that as a child the patient had been very constipated, and that from very early infancy his mother had been in the habit of giving him enemas per rectum to relieve this condition, and he remembered that he grew to like this operation and saw that in his infantile mind it had taken on in a disguised form something of the nature of a sexual act between his mother and himself. This was reinforced at a later date by the fact that when he was ill a hospital nurse gave him enemas, and in this instance he stated that his sexual pleasure was not even disguised. He had phantasies as a boy as to how he would have to look after his mother when his father died (his father was twenty-five years older than his mother), and he made up his mind that he would certainly not marry if it in any way interfered with his filial duty. Gradually he also came to identify himself with his mother, and when she became ill he took upon himself all the household details and the ordering of the servants. When she died, he transferred

* *Folie du doute.* See footnote on page 84.

his fixation to a sister, and insisted to me that he was going to take the part of a mother towards her and see that she did not miss her mother— this in spite of the fact that his father was alive, that his aunt came to act as housekeeper, and that there was no need for him continually to worry his head about household duties, which he did daily to such an extent that he had not at the time made any effort to earn his living in any profession. His dreams were strongly homosexual and anal-erotic, except when they were obviously sexual dreams towards the mother and sister, these occuring several times a week.

Case 3.—A woman whose father went abroad soon after her birth, and whose fixation was first of all upon the mother, showed a strong fixation on the mother in which she played the *masculine* part in the unconscious. At the age of two she again went to live with her father and developed a strong fixation upon him : but *she was still playing the male role*, and this time towards her father, so that we have the curious complex of a woman's fixation upon a man being of a homosexual nature.* This is accounted for by the fact already stated that everyone is bisexual, and that the actual sexual

*This reversal of the sexual rôle gives us an inkling into the formation of so called "invert homo-sexuality." I have recently had a male patient who showed a similar complex.

feelings in the reproductive organs of a woman are masculine in character. The aggressive and masculine part of her sexuality was already developed somewhat before her fixation on the father was formed : therefore she unconsciously acted the part of the male. She afterwards married a man who had many attributes similar to those of her father and towards whom she was sexually anæsthetic. In many of her dreams she showed strong *homosexual* fixation towards her *husband*, in which dreams she was in masculine clothes, and her husband was dressed as a priest in long robes, etc. For obvious reasons, I do not feel justified in giving further details of this interesting case, as her psychoneurosis was of a peculiar character, and the patient would readily be recognised by those who know her.

Case 4.—A woman of thirty-eight had a strong fixation on the father to whom as a child she used to go with all her little troubles and was petted and spoiled by him. Towards her mother she felt antagonism : as a child she felt that her mother never understood her and that she could never have taken her troubles to her mother. Her father died when she was sixteen years old, and her compulsion neurosis began shortly afterwards. In her early adult life she was in love with several men, all of whom were strangely like her father in type. Finally she married a man the exact reverse of her father in almost every respect both mentally and physically, showing that her incest complex was too near consciousness to permit her to marry the father type. However, in spite of her having married the reverse of the father type, in her unconscious the husband still represented the father, and towards him she had sexual anæsthesia. From a profound sense of duty she took her mother to live with her always (the result of the feeling of guilty jealousy in younger days) and she was continually quarrelling with her mother, who tried to rule the household. Love and hate were always at war with one another in her towards her mother for over twenty years, during which time the compulsion neurosis persisted with fluctuations. Amongst other things she related that soon after her father's death her mother took her to sleep with her in the same bed, and during the night wanted to be affectionate with her, putting her arms round her and so forth. The girl, however, had strongly resented this, and could not bear her mother to touch her and used to make excuses for lying as far away from her as possible. As the analysis progressed the patient had frequent dreams of incestuous relations with the father and of wishes to get rid of the mother.

Even twenty-two years after the father's death
she on one occasion had an emotional
breakdown in which she trembled violently and
wept simply because the idea had occurred to
her of how upset her father would be did he
know of the unhappiness her neurosis had caused.
The analysis of this case was interesting from
another point of view—namely, that the handing
on of psychoneuroses in families, as I have
previously pointed out, is not so much a question
of heredity as of early training and environment.
In this case the mother was highly neurotic
and had a mild neurosis somewhat similar to the
daughter's. The mother herself had a strong
father fixation and had married a father substitute towards whom her sexual life was inadequate, both for herself and for her husband.
As a consequence the husband projected too
great a proportion of affection and erotic
feeling upon his daughter, who in his unconscious
to a great extent supplied the affection he felt
was lacking towards him from his wife : the
result of this was that the daughter again obtained a father complex of undue proportions,
and unless care be taken or an analysis is made
of her own daughter, still a small child, the
neurosis will again for the same reason be handed
on, signs of it being already apparent.

One or two instances from Brill I should like

to quote, because although those I have mentioned are to the analyst perfectly obvious they have not the outstanding features which appeal to the beginner, who but vaguely realises the facts.

" A very cultured man was attracted only by very stout servants. No other type of woman appealed to him. Analysis showed that his first sexual impulses were aroused by a servant girl of that type who took the place of his mother."

" A refined married woman of twenty-four years suffered from psychosexual frigidity, but was sexually excited whenever she saw a lame man. This was due to an identification with her mother who had an illicit love affair with a man when the daughter was three or four years old. Like a great many grown-ups her mother considered her little girl an unthinking being and took no pains to conceal anything from her. When her paramour sustained a fracture of his leg and she found it necessary to make frequent calls on him she took her little daughter with her so as to avoid gossip. Although what she witnessed apparently made no impression on her at the time it nevertheless acted as a sexual trauma and formed an association between sex and lameness. This was also determined by the fact that at a later age this lame man took the place of her own father by marrying her widowed mother."

" A young married woman, dominated by a veritable prostitution complex, carried on illicit relations with men while she lived with her husband. Psycho-analysis showed that she was an only daughter and although her father's pet she saw very little of him during her early childhood as his affairs took him away from home. As far as her memory reached she recalled witnessing unholy loves between her mother and " strange men." She herself married a man who not only belongs to the same type as her father, but who even follows her father's vocation. She thus identified herself with her mother in every respect." *

* Brill; *Psychanalysis : its theory and practical application.*

CHAPTER VI

NARCISSISM

Narcissism is the term applied to that complex whose chief attribute consists in self-worship or self-admiration. We are not dealing with the conscious self-worship, such as may be seen in any auto-sexual exhibitionist, but with something much more subtle, much more disguised, and primarily at any rate much less erotic. For the narcissistic complex takes its early foundations in the pre-erotic stages of development, as we shall see immediately in considering its development.

We cannot suppose that the psychic life of the child commences only on the date of its birth. Just as *in utero* its heart beats. and it may move its little limbs, so no doubt in the unconscious it is laying the foundation of future mentality, and registering in some measure the effect of various stimuli which reach it *in utero*, *e.g.*, movement and sound.

Let us briefly examine its position here and through the changes that precede and follow birth.

Previous to birth, had it any conscious imagining at all it would naturally suppose itself to be the only individual in existence, moreover it would be an all-powerful individual. It does no work, it makes no effort, yet it is kept warm, it is fed, it is sheltered from every possible ill. In fact all its " life-desires " or unconscious wishes are fulfilled and kept in a condition of continual fulfilment.

Now let us see what happens at birth. Its peaceful omnipotence is rudely disturbed as it is forced down a narrow tunnel and out into the cold world. It feels its first pain. It takes its first breath, *it has to make its first effort to adjust itself to reality*. But it is not required to make a very great effort. Hardly has it made its first few cries, than it finds that all becomes well again. The nurse wraps it up warmly and places it again near the mother. Its previous warm, safe position is returned to it as far as possible.

During the first few days this procedure is repeated with slight variations. It cries—it is fed. It cries—and it is rocked gently to sleep (as it was " rocked " *in utero* by the mother's movements).* It cries—and a crooning song, a lullaby is hummed over it just as the lullaby of extra uterine sounds must have reached it previously. It curls up and sleeps. In other words when the child cries it finds it can magically and at once satisfy all its desires. True it has to cry, but otherwise its omnipotence is but little disturbed. All the world that it knows moves at its feeble cry to give it satisfaction and a semblance of its mother's womb.

This goes on for several months of the infant's life, but during that period the normal child is made to come gradually into contact with the realities of life, and to discover that all things do not belong to it nor are they all conducive to its pleasures. Upon the age to which this disillusionment is put off depends largely the future powers of adaptation of the child.

It is obvious that the new born infant lives in a world of *phantasy* in which the relative importance of itself and of things outside itself is not merely distorted but is entirely absent, and if we could suppose a child kept artificially in this condition to adult life, every wish satisfied instantaneously, every force it knows directed entirely to gratifying its immediate desire, not much imagination is needed to understand how absolutely lost this omnipotent creature would be on suddenly being turned into the world to face life and reality. His one desire would be to attempt to return to his omnipotent state, his one effort to keep at bay *reality* and turn it into the pleasant phantasy of the previous

twenty years. For he would surely before his
disillusionment have really come to believe
himself omnipotent, the only real thing in a
world of his own fashioning and dreaming.

An extreme case of this kind is of course an
impossibility, but there are varying degrees in
which it is approached, *if the infant be allowed to
postpone its acquaintance with reality too long,
it becomes " fixed " in a more or less degree in its
condition of phantasy.*

It is then said to have a strong narcissistic
fixation, or complex.

In all persons this is present in some degree.
Each one regards himself as the most real thing
present, though but few carry it far enough to
imagine that all others are merely part of a
dream in which the dreamer is the only real
figure, as the Red King, in " Alice through the
Looking Glass " is supposed to have done, when
the remark is made, " You're only a sort of
thing in his dream ! If that there King was
to wake, you'd go out—bang !—just like a
candle."

The effects of the narcissistic complex are
however very apparent in many people, and
have much to do with many of the psychoneurotic conditions. Among the simpler and more
common characteristics caused by it we find
impatience, the desire to accomplish something

at the instant of the conception of the wish, even at the expense of future pain. There is a lack of ability to count the cost, for in the unconscious that individual is all-powerful and able to avert further unpleasant consequences.

While at first narcissism is not concerned with erotic emotions, being pre-infantile-erotic in origin, it is nevertheless sooner or later connected with the infantile erotic impulses as would naturally be expected, but it must not be confused with auto-sexuality as is so often the case. One of the erotic channels into which narcissism often turns is homosexuality. We have discussed this hitherto as being largely determined by parental fixations, it is time now however, to modify this somewhat ; for just as the narcissistic person unconsciously regards himself as the one real and important individual, so he fails to admire anything in others which is not like himself, and he or she will be likely to have strong erotic feelings towards some member of the same sex having outstanding characteristics of himself.

If it does not proceed to this extent, the love-object on a hetero-sexual plane will probably be as near the individual's own physical or mental type as possible. Moreover, the narcissist will have considerable contempt for members of the opposite sex, as a rule, and tend to regard them as fundamentally and by Nature's design below him (or her) in the scale of creation.

One sees therefore that narcissistic and parental complexes are interdependent forces in the formation of the love-object of the individual.

The narcissistic individual may be quite happy and contented as long as the facts which he has to face are not too great for him to overcome, *i.e.*, as long as he remains in undisturbed possession of his " omnipotent idea ; " and since he almost invariably dismisses future trouble from his mind, *and hence is able to deal with it when it arises as a single isolated incident*, he is often able to achieve great things in a spasmodic way, and to live as an optimist, for he does not grasp any picture of disaster— nothing of that kind is real, he only is real. However, should his power be insufficient to overcome the difficulties that arise, the result may be unfortunate for him.

In the first place, as with any other complex of unbearable ideas which is repressed, a psychoneurosis may result. More commonly however a *regression*, or attempt to get back to childhood and omnipotence may take place in other ways. He may become a chronic alcoholic, for by means of alcohol the unpleasant reality is made to disappear ; he again becomes omnipotent. Under the influence of alcohol he also loses his sense of responsibility, and is mentally in the same irresponsible condition as when his mother nursed him and looked after him, *i.e.*, the condition of omnipotence when all his wishes were fulfilled.* Drug-taking is often a regression due to the same cause.

On the other hand the patient may seek other modes of regression. He may begin to cry like a baby, for as a child he found his tears were omnipotent in overcoming his difficulties. He may seek refuge in sleep (pathological bed-lying) for here once again he has reached the infantile omnipotence. He may fall into a rage and stamp and shout, for so at one period by means of such magic gestures did he gain from his parents obedience to his omnipotent will. Or again narcissists may become merely miserable, pessimistic persons who complain of everything and everyone, and are quite unable to adjust themselves to the new unpleasant reality, so unlike their previous dreams and ideals.

Many narcissistic persons complain of a lack of reality in life, and on occasion may even state that objects around them do not seem real, and that they can sometimes scarcely bring themselves to consider them as real.

*Alcoholism acts as a means of partially destroying repression in many other cases, and in particular in the complexes of homo-sexuality and exhibitionism.

It will be seen then how important is the behaviour of parents towards their children in the first few months of life. Not only as regards preventing a too-strong erotic fixation, but from the point of view also of preventing a too-strong narcissistic fixation. The two sets of complexes are often found strongly developed side by side as is to be expected, but since narcissism is pre-sexual and considerably earlier in its formation than the Œdipus complex, we find it more pronounced in certain cases. For instance an " *only* " child is very frequently not only narcissistic but has a very strong Œdipus complex ; whereas an *eldest* child may have an equally strong narcissistic complex also but a more normal Œdipus complex, since though the parents were his willing servants when he was a novelty, yet when the second child came eighteen months later, they were educated to a more sensible régime, and moreover since there were now two children they could no longer devote the same time and worship to the first. It is probable that the old idea of the inheritance of the eldest son, and of his other rights over the remaining members of the family, follow from his own narcissistic delusions brought about by his parents and afterwards thrust upon the world by himself from time immemorial.

CHAPTER VII

PRINCIPLES OF THINKING

REMARKS on this subject follow naturally on our study of Narcissism, in which we have seen how individuals may live largely in phantasy if they are unable to adapt themselves to reality. Methods of thought have been divided by certain psychologists into two main types with various subsidiary forms, and the nomenclature of these is somewhat involved. For our purposes they may, however, be reduced to

(1) Phantasy thinking (day-dreams, etc.) ;
(2) Directive thinking (reality thinking).

1. *Phantasy Thinking*.—We have seen how the Narcissist, unable to adapt himself to or even to realise the significance of, his surroundings, dwells in a world inside himself—a world in which in extreme cases he is himself the omnipotent ruler. We shall see in a future chapter on Dreams how the infantile mind satisfies itself with creating a similar world of its own. If the child cannot obtain all its desires, it will imagine that it has done so and

get satisfaction from this day-dream or phantasy instead of from reality. For instance, a child desires a pony to ride ; lacking this, a chair with a piece of string tied to it, or even a picture of a pony in a book will suffice as the object round which phantastic journeys over mountain and plain group themselves—the pleasure being unobtainable in reality is obtained in phantasy. It will be observed, however, that *these thoughts produce no effect on the outer world and lead to no action.* While the child travels 10,000 miles in imagination he has been sitting on the floor in reality.

Phantasy thinking is not always quite so simple as this. It is often, especially in hysterical subjects, combined with what is known as *identification.* We have already shown how strong is the influence of the parents on the child in forming our Oedipus complex. On to this other complexes may be grafted. It is by no means uncommon for a child to be brought up to look upon his father as one of the greatest of men, while he himself is impressed with the fact of his smallness and his incapacity for ever becoming so great as his father. Now we have shown that in the infantile mind this child has to some extent already fixed himself upon the mother, and the father is thus a rival in his unconscious mind. The rivalry now causes, in the natural course of events, some self-comparison with his father. It is possible that he feels that never will he succeed in attaining the exaggerated greatness with which his father is credited, and, just as naturally, he falls into a habit of acquiring in day-dreams those powers which he never hopes to obtain in reality. And in the unconscious there is much necessity for this, because, as his father's rival, he can never hope to obtain a position in his mother's heart equal to his father's, unless he can show those qualities which he assumes, and rightly, are in a large measure responsible for his mother having been attracted to the father. He thus, unconsciously perhaps, copies his father's mannerisms, method of speech, faults as well as virtues, and comes to a great extent to *identify himself with his father*.

This is by no means the only process by which identification may take place. A Narcissistic person very readily identifies himself with a large number of people in turn on somewhat the following lines. He sees in himself the only real and important personage : in progressing through the world he comes into contact with a new type, we will say, which expresses one of his own ideals far better than he does himself. He may at once identify himself with that person, and in imagination express himself in a similar manner. For instance, let us say our Narcissist has strong exhibition tendencies, but does not succeed because of external inhibitions in presenting himself sufficiently before the notice of the rest of the world. He goes to the theatre and sees an eminent actor occupying the centre of the stage, gazed at and applauded by all. On reaching home he immediately has phantasies in which he takes the place of this actor, grows tall and comely, has the grand manner, and in phantasy occupies the public eye. He has begun to identify himself with the actor in question.

There are many other ways in which identification with somebody else may take place in the unconscious. A person with an extremely strong fixation on, say, the mother, may come to identify himself gradually with her. I have already quoted a case in which a youth identified himself with his mother, and when she died insisted on taking her place in the household in almost every detail.

Now in phantasy thinking this question of identification plays an important part. When we read a novel we feel all the emotions of the hero or heroine, and at times feel such sympathy that we may even weep. What has been the cause of this? We have in fact been living through a day-dream, travelling through places and encountering adventures and experiences which are not open to us in real life, in the person of the hero or heroine .with whom we have identified ourselves. The author, of course, has himself done the same, and hence all novelists are largely phantasy thinkers. It is the same with poetry or with a play. Overwhelming sympathy with someone in trouble is again a question of identification; we put ourselves in his place and we feel his feelings.

In hysterical patients this identification and phantasy thinking combined are extremely noticeable. A hysterical patient will often identify himself in turn with almost everyone with whom he is brought into contact.

In everybody there is of course a certain amount of this phantasy thinking, and there seems to be no reason why a strictly limited amount should not be indulged in. It is a form of rest, and rest is needed by everyone. We may look upon sleep as a Narcissistic regression—a return to the condition of pre-birth. We may look upon a small amount of phantasy thinking in much the same light. But it is as dangerous to indulge in as morphia. As a habit it grows; as a habit it is extremely deleterious, because phantasy thinking, *i.e.*, undirected think ing, cannot take place simultaneously with directed or reality thinking,, and it is this latter

which is important to the formation of every
character, in the acquirement of every habit,
in the essntial progress of the world.

2. *Directive Thinking.*—Directive thinking
may be defined as that form of thinking which
has as its object *definite change.* The change
may be external to the thinker, a change produced in the world, either in its happiness, its
morals, its commercial prosperity or in other
forms of progress or deterioration, or perhaps,
more generally it may be a change affecting the
individual's own happiness or prosperity, or it
may be directed towards a mental change in the
thinker himself without his having any immediate idea of changing his external surroundings.
For instance, a man may wish to improve his
own character with regard to a bad habit.   He
does this perhaps by giving himself auto-suggestion or by thinking carefully and analysing
the causes of his habit with a view to eradicating
it.   All this, even though a change in the individual may not apparently take place, may be
classed as directive thinking. Directive thinking is thus obviously *controlled thinking, requiring
an effort of attention and concentration, whereas
phantasy thinking is for the most part uncontrolled.*   In all the business of everyday life
directive thinking must be employed, whether
we are merely deciding upon the position in

which to put the bulbs in the garden or whether
we are deciding upon the policy to be pursued
in a great commercial enterprise. Every time
we use our brains in directive thinking we are
establishing a habit which gradually gives us
power to produce changes in our environment
and in the world in general. Every time we
indulge in phantasy thinking we are encouraging
the habit of living in a world of our own ideas
and we are destroying the habit which enables
us to create. The two forms of thinking may
of course overlap considerably. The novelist
or the poet, for instance, are largely phantasy
thinkers : they feel the emotions of the various
characters which they evolve, but they have to
use directive thinking in order to arrange the
words and the sentences and furthermore they
may have the more distant aim of portraying
to the world an ideal or of drawing attention to
some evil and of suggesting their own remedy.
All this may have involved highly intensified
directive thinking.

It is obvious then that directive thinking need
not merely apply to things of the immediate
present or near future, and in trying to draw a
distinction between the two one is often con-
fronted with the superficial criticism that certain
ideas must pertain to phantasy thinking " because they will never come to pass."   The mere

possibility, however, that a thing may come to pass in two or three hundred years' time, for instance, and that the thoughts which have led to the production of the distant aim have been carefully sorted and weighed, constitutes those thoughts as directive.

If the average man sat in his arm-chair and thought out a wonderful plan for the conquest of Europe without having either the will or the means to carry out his ambitions, that would constitute phantasy thinking, but if Napoleon did the same, with the will and possible means, with a near aim at hand in the conquest of a small country and the far possibility in mind as an ultimate aim, we should have present direct-ive thinking; so that similar thoughts in two different individuals might really be classified under two different principles of thinking.

We have already pointed out how in every individual there appears to be a given amount of psychic energy. Now it is obvious that the more energy is expended upon phantasy think-ing the less there will be available for directive thinking. Hence from the point of view of energy expenditure it is again obvious how essential it is to cultivate deliberately the right form of thinking, once one has recognised one's deficiencies in this respect; and one of the greatest helps which any individual can have in doing this is to consider what *aim* he has in life. Most people will find on self-examination that their aim is by no means clearly defined. It is often merely a question of somehow getting through life with enough food to eat and enough phantasy thinking to keep them from boredom. This is especially the case with women whose household duties may require but little thought. Dusting a table becomes a habit which is most easily accompanied by phantasy thinking, whereas had that woman had some definite aim, apart from the mere *habit* of house-cleaning, it would be possible to accompany the table-dusting with directive thought which revolved round the aim in question.

If a person on self-examination finds that his aim or aims are not clearly defined, or on the other hand that his aims in themselves are phantasies and impossible of fulfilment, it were better that that person should at once deliberately remould and state his aims so that they become

(a)   clearly defined ;

(b)   clearly possible.

Moreover, aims should be of two kinds :—

(1)   Immediate ;

(2)   Remote.

The remote aim is the ideal towards which we are striving, and it should be possible of fulfilment—(not necessarily in our lifetime in all cases).

The immediate aim should always be in harmony with the remote aim.

Phantasy thinking not only wastes psychic energy in itself, but, if encouraged, may be very deleterious in leading to the development and persistence of various infantile erotic impulses, and, *vice versa*, certain of such impulses may lead to phantasy thinking. Thus we get a vicious circle. For instance, an individual with highly developed phantasies, with but little of his energy devoted to the realities of life, will very likely (from the same causes which first induced this condition) be prone to masturbation. The less energy he puts into directive thinking, and the more he becomes accustomed to fulfilling his wishes in the form of phantasies, the more is this likely to be the case. Masturbation is nearly always connected with some form of phantasy in which the masturbation plus the phantasy represent a heterosexual (or homosexual) act. For instance, the imagination of the individual first contemplates the beautiful wife (or husband) in a day-dream : he proceeds through courtship and marriage in phantasy, and with the help of masturbation he finally completes the picture. Afterwards, if he by some effort breaks himself of the habit he may be liable to an anxiety hysteria, such as is described in a later chapter, in which phantasy, now displaced into another sphere, again plays an important part. *Vice Versa*, if the ıct of masturbation be started without phantasy it will almost inevitably tend to produce one in its early stages and thus encourage the vicious circle.

Practically all other infantile impulses and aims may in a similar way be intermingled with phantasy thinking, to the detriment of the individual.

Apart from the obviously erotic side of phantasy thinking many would say : " But my greatest pleasure is to be found in daydreams. I find in directive thinking nothing but hard work." Obviously, in such a case, if the individual cannot enjoy his directive thinking, *i.e.*, gets no emotional discharge by means of it, some sort of analysis might be useful in assisting him. For what he really needs for his phantasy thinking is sublimation, exactly as he needs this for many of his infantile erotic impulses. It is probable that this individual's aim is not one suited to him, in which case subsidiary aims should be formed wherein an interest in directive thinking could be taken. He will then find an emotional outlet in the result of this directive thinking and will more easily decrease the time devoted to phantasy thinking.

Some sublimation may, however, be found in certain forms of phantasy thinking. For instance, Pfister states with truth : " It is certain that phantasy thinking can bring about a great spiritualisation and deepening of the emotional life in a good sense, but it is equally certain that in the over-emphasis of this phantasticism, which would offer a substitute for a deficiency in reality, an immense amount of noble strength is lost to reality. . . With the neurotic the role of the wish phantasy is much greater than with the normal individual. He puts his whole life force into it. He solves the problems which life imposes on him by a phantasy, for every neurotic phenomenon is only the automatic realisation of such a phantasy. It is therefore quite correct for him to esteem an unallowed phantasy as highly as an act. To many the phantastic activity is so dear that they would rather endure the severest suffering than part with it."*

It is obvious from the foregoing that in all phantasy thinking we have the fulfilment of a wish, and in this respect dreams, hysterias and phantasies are alike, and, for a similar reason, phantasies are of great value in psycho-analysing any patient.

* Pfister: " Psycho-analytic Method."

Even from the type of book that a person reads one may judge fairly clearly some of his complexes. If a child possesses the passion for reading it may be judged from this standpoint. " This phenomenon always occurs only in children whose demands for love mastery or execution are too little gratified in reality . . . "

" . . . From the kind of reading preferred a skilled educator can at once see what kind of unsatisfied longing `exists in the young bookworm : whether love, hunger or hate, sadism, (detective novels), or desire for recognition. Even plans for invention often form a bit of automatism. Behind the aviatistic endeavours of boys there often exists that erotic desire which also manifests itself with extreme frequency in dreams of flying. If one forbids such automatisms without providing something better one blocks up a harmless, indeed, in certain circumstances, useful outlet, while by means of analysis the condition is often easily corrected and fundamentally improved. . . The task of the analyst therefore very often consists in guiding back the pleasure-seeking automatist (phantasy thinker) from his ' private theatre,' his ' cloudland ' and gaining his life energy for humanity and productive ends."*

Inertia is the common (superficial) cause of

* Pfister : Psycho-analytic Method : p. 310.

most phantasy thinking. The majority of educated people, of so-called normal type, when they have completed their day's work, are fatigued, and can work no more without some sort of mental rest. And some kind of phantasy thought is resorted to. When this is cumulative they say : " We have worked eleven months and require one month's holiday." This is really merely an unconscious phantasy requiring a *regressive* reward. Even in these people the idea of *rest*, which often means undirected thought, holidays with no effort, etc., forms the ideal at the end of a year's strenuous labour. But it must be borne in mind that there is yet a higher type in whom the ideal still remains directive thought : a change in immediate aim rather than a phantasy forms their holiday or rest period."

Phantasy thinking such as we have already discussed in principle may take many other surreptitious forms which are not commonly so thought of. In old age that feeble type known to all, which is slipping into a thoughtless imbecility, is the same type which at an earlier stage of life has lacked directive thoughts ; on the other hand, our intellectual old man or old woman, still full of the day's problems and politics, is one who indulged but little in early phantasies. Experience shows us that the influence of directed or undirected thought in youth may not only determine our happiness in declining years but the actual age to which we live.

Even now we have not completely discriminated between directed and undirected thought. A casual conversation between acquaintances in which no information of importance is imparted, in which merely some emotional material is brought to the surface, is undirected thought. The first person with an unsatisfied emotional experience retails to the second person the facts of that experience, but as a rule without arousing an emotional experience in the second person. Such conversation is commonly known as " small talk." It takes place over the vast majority of afternoon tea-tables ; it is waste energy ; it is undirected thinking ; it is part of our organised present condition of semi-civilization, and, it is deleterious not only to the State but to the individual, not only to the individual but to the State. Another example is that of letter writing in certain instances. The letter—the duty letter —which must conventionally be written, is of the same calibre. The writer who deals with his or her experiences on a summer holiday or a shopping excursion, whichever it be, to the utter boredom of the recipient, is merely again expressing phantastic, undirected thoughts. There is no return for the expended energy. The rush of ideas produces no result. The emotion is insincere and conveys nothing but a conventional interest. It is time for a letter to be written; it is the "turn" for that letter to be written, and phantasy thinking is a result of the boredom and emptiness of the present conventional conditions. The writer of such a letter will often be observed to be biting the end of his or her pen while thinking out the contents. This is not the meaningless act it seems. It is a regression. He is performing an act ruinously expensive to himself. He is taking a Narcissistic nourishment from a mother pen. He is demonstrating the misdirected levelopment of his unconscious.*

I have already shown how in reading a novel our interest is a form of phantasy thinking in which we identify ourselves with the hero, and the same occurs in our theatres and in our cinematograph shows, (in the latter by the pleasures of enhanced phantasy thinking, *i.e.*, the real-visual, not merely the word-visual). These are within reach of anybody possessing a few pence ; and although the average person may regard them as educational and useful to the community, the magistrate who is dealing with a youthful delinquent knows the cinematograph influence to be harmful to the child mind. There is no doubt that the psychological effect of such

* Lay: Man's Unconscious Conflict.

mental stimuli is exceedingly deleterious to the race in general. The indulging in them encourages the habit of phantasy thinking at small cost, and such a habit becomes established as a part of the individual make-up. Like dreams, like hysterias, the scenario is but the phantastic wish-fulfilment of the spectator or reader. Nor does the evil stay itself here. The phantasy is the fulfilment of impossible wishes in these cases, and the emotional output is increased out of all proportion to the real exciting causes; this results in a misplacement of the emotional output in the unconscious mind, which in its turn is a basis of many neurotic conditions. And one must remember that a neurotic condition may not merely be an illness in an individual—it may be, and often is, the disease of a nation.

It is therefore obvious that the mental health of the individual and of the nation may be preserved by retaining in consciousness the reality of everyday life and of each isolated situation, whether the matter be painful or pleasurable.

Phantastic thought always implies (or nearly always) the repression into the unconscious of all directive thinking that is giving pain : it is the avoidance of facts with an unrealisable replacement.

In childhood this can be co ibated or encouraged. The fairy tale is commonly regarded
as the infant's prerogative : it is really, in spite
of popular prejudice, the infant's bane.
" What," says the reader, " would my little
boy be without his fairy tale ? I tell him one
every evening." Every evening, let me repeat,
you are encouraging him to avoid the real facts
of life and to substitute phantasies which in later
life will cause many tears to flow. Even in
childhood let there be a sublimation in displacement of energy. The child can obtain pleasure
by directive thinking which entails building
with bricks, tearing up paper, anything con-
structive or destructive and preferably the
former, as much and even more than by the
mere phantasy of the fairy tale or the punishment of the bogie ; though these may displace
energy, may satisfy the infantile artistic idea
of enjoyment, they lead nowhere except to
mental deterioration.

CHAPTER VIII

DREAMS

A DREAM is not a senseless medley of thoughts, as has been generally supposed ; it has a very perfect mechanism with a very definite meaning and object. So much is this the case that the dream becomes an invaluable aid in psycho-analysis : indeed, without the dream, in most cases, we could not carry out a psycho-analysis at all thoroughly.

Although Freud recognises only one type of dream, I myself definitely recognise three; I do not hesitate to say, however, that over 99 per cent of all dreams are of the Freudian type. The important (Freudian) dream I will discuss last of all, as practically the whole of this chapter will be devoted to this type. The other two types, though rare, appear to me very definite. They scarcely enter into psycho-analysis : but in order to give here a comprehensive study of dreams as they have come under my notice these types must have their place in this chapter. I will deal with them briefly, then, before passing on to the Freudian dream.

Type 1.—Of this type is the dream in which some past event of a horrible nature recurs positively without disguise and in all its detail. This may or may not cause the individual to waken according to the amount of energy behind its content. This type of dream refers always to incidents in which the actual preservation of life itself appeared threatened. Here, probably, there is a pent up emotion of fear, and the dream is possibly an attempt to work off this emotion of fear (abreaction). In ordinary life this type of dream appears but rarely ; it has, however, come to my notice extremely frequently in soldiers suffering from neuroses following experiences in the war. These dreams will be mentioned later in connection with anxiety neuroses.

Type 2.—This type of dream, which is extremely rare, is telepathic. Here the dreamer sees in his dream some actual happening which is taking place, or has taken place, at a distance. I have recently investigated several instances of this which seem to leave the fact beyond doubt. However, except for the interest connected with this type of dream and its possibilities, we shall find no useful purpose served by a study of it here, and we shall let this brief mention of it suffice for the present.

Type 3.—In order to make clear the importance of this third and usual type of dream we must again refer at some length to our constant habit of repression. It will be remembered that from childhood upwards social and ethical conditions have been forcing us to repress the majority of our primitive desires; and this by no means refers only to erotic desires. The child sees a kitten in a neighbour's house—he immediately desires to possess it; he sees cakes and chocolates on the table, and endeavours at once to make them his own. In early infancy there is no instinct of repression; the infant's mind is absorbed by a variety of wishes, and he attempts to gratify them all at once. Now if each child were not trained to repress desires of this kind, life would be intolerable for all. No society, even of the most barbaric and primitive form, could exist. We should be attempting to possess ourselves of other people's property, wives and so forth. Consequently, unless we lived absolutely alone and at war with the rest of mankind, existence would be impossible. Hence, very rightly, we must from childhood upwards repress our insatiable desires. If one stops to consider them for a moment it will be seen that though our desires are manifold *it is a fact that few of them are ever attained.*

Let us now see what happens to the child when repression first begins to take place. If he cannot have a real pony he contents himself with a rocking horse ; failing this, he will amuse himself by tying toy reins to another child and imagining that the other child is the pony ; failing this again, he will sit in a chair and vividly imagine the delights of driving a horse— he will see himself manipulating a coach and four or careering over desolate mountains on a fiery untamed steed : *in other words, he obtains satisfaction of his desire by means of a day dream or phantasy.* This process goes on to a certain extent throughout the whole life of each individual, but as we grow older so do we generally gain satisfaction of our desire, not by a day dream but by turning the energy of the desire into another channel, through which it may flow to more advantage, *i.e.*, we sublimate the energy into something which is legitimate and possible, and instead of dreaming of those things which are unattainable and trying to gain satisfaction from a day dream *we learn to face and to deal with facts.*

Nevertheless, as we said before, in dealing with erotic desires the whole of our energy is never completely sublimated. There is always an unsatisfied *repression* striving for *expression* from the unconscious mind. Moreover, even in dealing with facts which are attainable, there is generally at the end of each day some un-accomplished or partially accomplished fact which still engrosses our conscious mind. We shall find that the ordinary dream weaves together the unaccomplished fact (legitimate desire) and the unsublimated wishes (repressed desires) and that these together form the dream.

We may formulate the main outlines of the dream, which we shall endeavour to illustrate later, as follows:

1stly.—It tends to preserve sleep by carrying on everyday conflicts of a disturbing nature under some form of disguise, *i.e.,* it prevents us from consciously considering our daily problems.

2ndly.—It serves as a means of obtaining the fulfilment of unattainable wishes.

3rdly.—If such wishes are of a nature foreign or loathsome to the conscious mind, it so disguises them as to prevent them from becoming conscious, and here again tends to preserve sleep.

When the dream is so constructed that it is unable to confuse and bear along the daily problem or to disguise the repressed and un-bearable wishes of the unconscious, then the dreamer finds the dream inacceptable and too vivid and wakes up.

In the infant the dream of the night is very
similar to the day dream. It has not yet learnt
to repress, nor has it yet developed its full
primitive sexuality in an acceptable condition ;
therefore we find but few disguised dreams.
Freud has divided the development of sexuality
into three main stages. Firstly, the primitive
forms of energy, that is, the sexual impulses.
This development takes place prior to the age
of four years, and may often result in actual
masturbatory acts considerably prior to this age.
The second period, which he designates as the
latent period is from about the age of four to the
age of eleven or thereabouts. During this
period, although the sexual impulses are each
developing, enormous repression is enforced by
ethical and social conditions, and such phenomena as infantile masturbation, and so forth, are
generally repressed. At or about the age of
eleven a third stage begins, when, owing to the
steady unconscious development of the sexual
impulses, the repression tends to break down,
and the sexual aim (*i.e.*, auto-, homo-, or heterosexuality) becomes more clearly differentiated,
though differentiation is not complete until
puberty.

. These three periods correspond with three
definite types of dream. The first period, in
which there is no repression, gives a type of

dream which merely discloses in an undisguised manner the unfulfilled wishes of the individual. The second period gives us a certain number of similar dreams, with others in which repressed erotic impulses occur, but in a more and more disguised form as the age advances. The third gives us dreams in which but few unfulfilled legitimate wishes are recognisable, and in which both repressed erotic impulses and erotic aims appear in the form of fulfilled wishes disguised so as not to shock the conscious judgment, the disguise being in proportion to the amount of repression. Unfulfilled desires, not of an erotic nature yet unpleasant to the conscious acceptance of things, also appear in a disguised form.

This then is the type of dream which we meet with in the ordinary individual every night, and with which we have to deal in psycho-analysis. Further, we have to assume for the purpose of gathering some idea of what takes place in the transformation of dreams that there is some intellectuality capable even in our sleep of recognising what would be unpleasant to our conscious mind. This is brought about by what may be termed the censor which may be regarded as standing between the conscious and the unconscious mind, and which so disguises the content of the dream that the accomplish-

ment of infantile wishes is quite unrecognisable
to the ordinary conscious mind. If this were
not the case, the following would happen :
when we slept and our primitive unconscious
mind with its perverse erotic wishes was no
longer controlled and subordinated by our
conscious mind, then our unconscious and brutal
instincts would obtain their gratification undisguised. The horror of these primitive wishes
would be so great that the dreamer would awake
frightened and disgusted, and it is only therefore
by very careful disguise of the content of the
dream that this horror is kept from consciousness, and incidentally, the sleep of the individual
preserved. Of the exact place or state of this
intellectuality we have not the remotest conception, but we are obliged to assume that it is there
because of the obvious work that is performed
in the dream, in the neurosis, and in the displacement of sexuality in everyday life ; and
we conveniently term this intellectuality the
" censor " of the unconscious, regarding it as
having a distinct individuality for the purpose
of gaining a clearer conception of its work.

  ʹ The dream is very similar to a cartoon in the
newspaper. A great statesman may one day
be represented as a crowing cock, on another
day as a rabbit, and on yet a third day as some
inanimate object in the cartoon. In the same

way in the dream the repressed material is disguised by various commonplace objects and happenings. Just as in the cartoon there is no absolute and finite standard of symbolism, so it is in the dream : the censor selects any odd material—a portion of which at any rate invariably comes from the happenings of the previous twenty-four hours, material which has not been thoroughly realised consciously—as the paint wherewith to colour his canvas. If blue is lacking to paint the sky in a Mediterranean scene he naïvely takes copper and lays the scene in the West Indies. The underlying plot, however, is in either case produced with fidelity.

But it must be remembered that *the emotions felt in a dream do not always correspond with the actual happenings in the dream, but with the ideas hidden behind the dream.* Thus one may fall off a cliff in a dream without experiencing any fear, because the symbolism of falling off a cliff in that particular dream represents nothing of a fearful nature ; whereas one might strike a match in a dream and have intense terror from apparently unexplained reasons—the real reason, however, being that the terror referred not to the striking of the match but to the idea which that action disguised.

Jung's conception of the work of dreams is

slightly different and involves the idea that the
dream reinforces conscience and so strengthens
one against the infantile wishes which are
expressed therein ; in other words, while Freud
looks upon the dream as determined entirely by
something which has gone before, Jung con-
siders that it is the conscience and that which is
coming after or raising the individual to a higher
ideal which influences the dream. He has
adduced no proof, whereas Freud has adduced
proof. Nevertheless, Jung may also be right,
the dream may also subserve other purposes
simultaneously, for there is no evidence *against*
his theory. I am personally inclined to a third
and more or less intermediate idea : my own
conception of dreams embraces Freud's work
entirely, but also adds that, as well as a primitive
infantile wish the sublimation thereof is expressed and attained ; and that that sublimation, even if never repeated in exactly the same
disguise, may, like other sublimations, become a
habit fixed in the unconscious. In other words,
there are at least two interpretations to many
dreams—one expressing the primitive wish and
the other the wish in a sublimated and higher
form. We have apparently an unconscious
instinct endeavouring constantly to guide us by
sublimating our primitive energy to a higher
type, and we must make a very clear distinction

between a sublimation and a displacement. For instance, suppose that a woman dreams that she is most wonderfully clothed, or even that she is walking the streets in nothing but her stockings. In either case we may have the primitive infantile exhibition wish. But supposing that in addition to being most wonderfully clothed she dreams that she has a halo on her head and a harp in her hands, we might be justified in assuming that we were here dealing with some type of sublimation in which a high moral rather than a high physical standard were the wish expressed. As a matter of fact we should find on analysis of this dream that *both* were expressed, but it would be obvious that moral sublimation is present as well as mere sexual displacement. Displacement is the earliest and crudest form of the struggle of the mind for a higher outlet, sublimation being a later and higher form. It is not my intention in this chapter to express an opinion of the origin of this tendency to the higher forms of sublimation.

Not all dreams nor all dreamers show sublimation in the dream work ; it is present in very varying amounts. But practically all dreams express the lower and primitive wishes, displace them and fulfil them, and a very large proportion show the added sublimation. The sublimation, moreover, frequently increases with the increased age of the individual.

A non-sexual but repressed wish is often expressed in the dream as well as the erotic wish above referred to. And since the same material is thus made to represent two distinct ideas, the dream may be spoken of as over-determined.

I will now quote one or two typical dreams, the meaning of which has been elicited from the patient under analysis by what is termed " free association." In this method the patient's attention is directed to any word or sentence in the dream, and he is told to give all the thoughts and ideas in connection with this word or sentence just as they come into his mind *without criticism and without repression.* The thoughts may be vulgar, personal, trivial, or they may be connected with other people's private affairs. Whatever they are, the patient *must* express them ; by this means we discover what lies behind, and what is connected unconsciously with any of the dream images. This will be much more fully explained when we consider the technique of psycho-analysis itself at a later stage. Let us commence our elucidation by means of an illustration outside dreams.

We will suppose that an artist has drawn a cartoon (=a dream) in which he has represented a cock with a large bent beak crowing on a rock surrounded by the sea. The artist drew this cartoon years ago, and has quite forgotten what it represented or when he drew it. We proceed somewhat as follows : *The Analyst :* " Give associations to the cock you see in the cartoon." *The Artist :* " A cocky fellow ; cock of the roost ; monarch of all he surveys. . . . a statesman who has got his own way comes into my mind. . . . He has got rather a beaky nose . . . . Gladstone comes into my mind. . " *Analyst :* " Now associations to the rock." *Artist :* " A useless sterile bit of land, not much to crow about ; an island in the sea. . . . I remember now ! Ireland, of course ! It was drawn on an occasion when Mr. Gladstone had made a triumphant speech on Home Rule, and I, not being much of a politician, thought it ' Much ado about nothing.' I thought that it did not really matter whether Home Rule were granted or not, considering that in any case Ireland, a thinly populated island cost us much more than she ever paid. It seemed to me a sterile rock so far as we were concerned."

The analysis, then, has brought from the unconscious to the conscious mind of the artist the original meaning of his cartoon.

Now supposing that instead of a cartoon by an artist this same scene had been described as a dream by Mr. Gladstone himself. The analysis might then by a similar process of free association have revealed the wish of Mr. Gladstone that his speech on Home Rule should result in his being " cock of the roost," or " monarch of all he surveyed," with reference to the conflict then being waged concerning Ireland. Moreover, the dream would not only have expressed his wish, it would have fulfilled it ; for in the dream he had taken up a commanding position on the rock, and this rock symbolised Ireland.

Now few dreams are so simple as the above example, for the simple reason that in order to disguise the feelings (especially when primitive erotic impulses are repressed, or when more than one wish is to be represented by the symbol, various artifices are resorted to by the censor. Moreover, it must be remembered that the censor is apparently obliged to make use of at least some material from the events of the twenty-four hours immediately preceding the dream. This will form the subject of his picture, but in order to disguise still more carefully the underlying feeling, he makes use of these further artifices :

1. *Displacement.*—By this we mean that the hidden content of the dream instead of being represented by the most prominent features

of the dream may be displaced and occupy a trivial position in the background. One's dream may consist apparently of a battleship ploughing the ocean, but the essential portion may lie behind a broken rope hanging over the side or a splash of rust upon one of the funnels.

2. *Condensation.*—A large number of factors bearing upon the wish expressed in the dream may be represented by one factor in the obvious content. Thus : if we wish to express envy towards a brother, a commercial rival, and a hypothetical devil simultaneously, we are quite likely to produce a composite figure of all three in one person, with the eyes of the brother, the moustache of the commercial rival and a lucifer match in his hands to indicate the devil, the result being quite unrecognisable to our conscious self, but which on analysis would be found to contain a large number of *condensed* ideas. Not only may personalities be combined, but a large series of experiences may be heaped together so as to reinforce one another, and be represented by only one simple image.

An excellent example of a dream containing much condensation is given by Ferenczi.* He says : " I was once called upon to analyse the very short dream of a woman ; in it she had wrung the neck of a little, barking, white dog.

* "Contributions to Psycho-Analysis," pp. 101-102.

She was very much astonished that she, 'who could not hurt a fly,' could dream such a cruel dream, and she did not remember having dreamt one like it before. She admitted that, being very fond of cooking, she had many times killed pigeons and fowls with her own hand. Then it occurred to her that she had wrung the neck of the little dog in the dream in exactly the same way as she was accustomed to do with the pigeons in order to cause them less pain. The thoughts and associations that followed had to do with pictures and stories of executions, and especially with the thought that the executioner, when he has fastened the cord about the criminal's neck, arranges it so as to give the neck a twist, and thus hasten death. Asked against whom she felt strong enmity at the present time, she named a sister-in-law, and related at length her bad qualities and malicious deeds, with which she had disturbed the family harmony, before so beautiful, after insinuating herself *like a tame pigeon* into the favour of her subsequent husband. Not long before a violent scene had taken place between her and the patient, which ended by the latter showing her the door with the words : ' Get out ; I cannot endure a biting dog in my house.' Now it was clear whom the little white dog represented, and whose neck she was wringing in the dream. The sister-in-law is also a small person, with a remarkably white complexion. This little analysis enables us to observe the dream in its displacing and thus disguising activity. Without doubt the dream used the comparison with the biting dog instead of the real object of the execution fancy (the sister-in-law) smuggling in a little white dog just as the angel in the Biblical story gave Abraham at the last moment a ram to slaughter, when he was preparing to slaughter his son. In order to accomplish this the dream had to heap up memory images of the killing of animals until by means of their condensed psychical energy the image of the hated person paled, and the scene of the manifest dream was shifted to the animal kingdom. Memory images of human executions served as a connecting link for this displacement.

" This example gives me the opportunity to repeat that, with few exceptions, the conscious dream content is not the true reproduction of our dream-thoughts, but only a displaced, wrongly accented caricature, the original of which can be reconstructed only by the help of psycho-analysis."

3. *Reduplication.*—By this we mean that certain points in the dream, or even complete wishes, may be represented by more than one

figure or symbol. Suppose, for instance, in the hypothetical dream above quoted concerning Mr. Gladstone reduplication had been present; we might have added to the cock crowing an enormous wave in the background overwhelming a boat, with a man in it whose face was similar to that of Salisbury, Gladstone's chief political opponent at that time, or there might have been a composite picture of all his opponents being overwhelmed by this wave. Here we should have had his triumph expressed twice in the same picture, and, from the point of view of a cartoonist, the second image would be superfluous. The wave would represent Mr. Gladstone in the same way as the cock does, so that the factors of the case would have been present twice over.

"If" and "an," "either" and "or" in a dream are expressed by simultaneous contrasts or consecutive happenings in time and space. The words themselves are absent from the picture.

It has been argued by many patients that the dreams they experience are occasionally diametrically opposed to their wishes, but even here it can be shown that it is not the expressed wish which counts; rather it is one implied by that apparent wish.

To illustrate this I cannot do better than

quote an excellent example which Brill has published.*

Relating the first dream he says : " Recently a patient came to me and disputed the theory of wish fulfilment. To prove his assertion he stated that the night before he had dreamed that he had syphilis. I could readily prove that the dream showed the realisation of a wish. This patient was being treated by me for psychic sexual impotence, and the day before his dream we discussed promiscuous sexuality. I called his attention to the dangers of infection, and spoke about proper precautions, etc. He grimly remarked : ' There is no danger of my becoming infected. I could not if I tried.' The dream realises his wish that he can become infected ; meaning that he is no longer sexually impotent. (Obviously the dream is not the wish that he should become infected, but that he should be in a position to be able to become infected)."

Patients frequently dream of the death of a parent or friend, and state that they cannot see how this can be a wish fulfilment. It is easy to demonstrate this to be the case, however. In dreams one frequently reverts to infantile modes of expression, indeed, some suppressed infantile material is practically always present in them. Now in infancy a child will often

* Psycho-Analysis : Its Theory and Practical Application,—Brill.

exclaim : " I wish you were dead ! " But he has no real conception of death ; he merely means : " I wish you were out of the way, you are interfering with my desires." And this is all that a death wish in a dream means on most occasions.

Dreams containing repressed infantile erotic wishes whose complexes have been " touched " during the day are extremely common in normal persons. For instance, I have frequently noticed that if a person has hæmorrhoids which suddenly irritate him the anal-erotic repressed impulse is touched, and the dream of the night will fulfil the wish connected with the anal-erotic impulse—quite disguised in as far as the patient is concerned, but often very obvious to the analyst even without analysis; and so with other repressed erotic impulses, which some trivial incident of the day has tended to bring nearer to consciousness.

A fact of considerable importance to the psycho-analyst is that dreams of the same night generally refer to the same complexes and that the second or third dreams are less disguised than the first, as though in repetition of the work the censor became careless and lost energy and hence was less able to disguise the wish effectively. ˟ An example of this is to be seen in the two following dreams which occurred in the same night to a woman patient,. one of whose symptoms was psycho-sexual impotence.

In the first dream she was riding a galloping horse ; at first she recalled no more, except that in the dream she felt very nervous. Later she added that she believed the horse had a short grey beard.

In the second dream she was mounting the stairs of a high tower with her father ; it was very difficult and her father had to help her ; at the top of the tower they both fell exhausted together.

The meaning of these two dreams was very obvious to me at once, but I naturally did not tell her so. Associations which she gave led to the following interpretation (which was the one I had already formed in my mind). The horse's beard resembled her father's beard. Her father had taught her to ride as a girl, and was very fond of horses of which he always had several. She had ridden with her father on the previous day (he was staying with her husband and herself). She said then that her father was a very " horsey " man and she then identified her father with the horse. She was " riding her father "—an obvious disguise for an incestuous erotic wish towards her father.

The second dream was at once quite obvious

to her then. In this dream the father was not even disguised; she was mounting the stairs with him and they fell exhausted together—an obvious symbol of the same erotic wish in the unconscious.

These dreams also show two rather typical symbols, riding and mounting stairs, and many other similar acts such as travelling in a motor boat, etc., which entail *regular rhythmic motion*, practically always represent a sexual act. And even in language the symbolism has been recognised, for the words "riding," "mounting," etc., have often been used to designate the same act.

As a matter of fact the reason of this patient's psycho-sexual impotence was that as an infant she had fallen in love with her father and *in her unconscious mind* had remained in that condition ever since and could not pass on the erotic energy to her husband. This, however has been much more fully discussed in the chapter on parental complexes.

There is of course no fixed symbolism in dreams, and symbols may represent one thing one day and another the next, but there are certainly several more or less typical symbols which, when present in a dream generally represent a given action or idea. We have already mentioned riding or mounting. Climbing a tree would be equally typical of the same act. Churches, boxes, etc., generally represent the female, often the mother idea, while elongated cylindrical things represent as a rule either the male reproductive organs or more rarely the female homologue of the same. Crossing a river or ravine generally indicates the successful accomplishment in the dream of overcoming some difficulty which has not been overcome in the waking life, and so forth. There is no need, however, to give examples of these dreams, as sufficient have already been given to demonstrate how dreams are formed, and their means of wish fulfilment.

SUMMARY

1. *The vast majority of dreams serve t͟o purposes : (a), the fulfilment of repressed or unattained wishes ; (b), the preservation of sleep.*
2. *The manifest content of the dream is formed from any material that lies handy, part of which comes from the events of the previous twenty-four hours.*
3. *The latent content, or inner meaning of the dream is disguised by the symbolism of the manifest content so as to be unrecognisable to the dreamer.*

4. *Part of the latent content always refers to infantile repressions.*
5. *The emotion in a dream has reference to the latent meaning and not to the manifest content.*

CHAPTER IX

The Functional Diseases

HYSTERIAS, anxieties and many other conditions of the mind follow naturally upon our discussions upon dreams, because what the dream is to the sleeper the nervous disease is to the waking life in many respects. The nightmare of sleep corresponds on the whole to the anxiety condition of the waking neurotic individual. In other words, the neurotic is living in a kind of dream. The most absurd dream may be quite real during sleep, *because it is split off from our conscious experience.* Thus a man may fall off a cliff 300 feet high in a dream and alight comfortably and without any sense of surprise in an armchair at the bottom of the cliff, because his conscious judgment about falling is split off from his dream experience. In hysteria a similar splitting of consciousness takes place. Our study of dreams, then, will have enabled us to understand much more readily our functional diseases. They are pathological conditions of the mind in which the absurdity of the situation as gauged by our

reasoning faculties is largely left in abeyance
—not by any deliberate and conscious effort,
but for the simple reason that our identity is
split into two or more portions, a gap lying
between the conscious and the unconscious
reasoning and conclusions, and this gulf remains
quite unbridgeable until analysed. This explanation applies to certain forms of hysteria
and lunacy: it does not apply equally to all
so-called functional diseases, for though some
of the functional diseases are occasioned by a
gap or a splitting off of consciousness in ideas
(ideals, memories, conflicts), others are the
result of accumulated *emotions* attendant upon
these ideas, and one must always remember
that the emotions are of a primary nature and
occur before any reasoning is applied thereto.
Thus while we may recognise that erotic
emotions connected with human beings follow
upon definite ideas of beauty or other attractions,
in our primitive ancestors we must recognise
emotions as something felt prior to deliberate
or reasoned ideas.   One cannot imagine that
the earthworm, an organism without eyes and
with ganglia representing the primitive brain,
has any particular ideas in connection with
another earthworm; but it can be imagined
that it has a compelling energy of emotion—
not connected with definite ideas—which causes

it to come into contact with another earthworm, to desire touch, and so forth, without a reasoned idea lying behind as motive.   There is, in other words, a stage in development in which emotions *per se* become emotions attached to a mental picture or idea.

We must therefore divide our psychic diseases into two classes : those connected with ideas with their attendant emotions, and those chiefly concerned with emotions themselves, whether in reality they have ideas attached to them or not.   Broadly speaking, the division is as follows :—

1. *The Psycho-Neuroses :* These are neurotic conditions following repressed ideas.
2. *The Actual Neuroses :* Those dependent upon accumulated emotions whether ideas are there in a subsidiary form or not.

The various neuroses have been classed by different writers in different ways ; this has been further complicated by the fact that they apparently overlap, and in overlapping form new combinations, which by superficial observers have been classified as new diseases.   Freud's classification is probably the most correct, and if I vary this slightly it is in order to simplify it from the point of view of the student, and not because the dogmatic classification which

I give is by any means final in its conception. My classification therefore, of the neuroses is as follows :—

1. *The Psycho-Neuroses* (the hysterias) :—
    a. Conversion Hysteria.
    b. Anxiety Hysteria.
    c. Compulsion Hysteria (compulsion neurosis).
    d. Paranoid Hysteria (early paranoia).
    e. Dementia Praecox (certain cases of).
2. *The Actual Neuroses :—*
    a. Anxiety Neurosis.
    b. Neurasthenia.

Here one must state that in spite of the separation of the actual neuroses from the psycho-neuroses we shall find later on that they overlap, for the anxiety hysteria and the anxiety neurosis have very much in common. Indeed, one might almost state that the anxiety neurosis is included in the anxiety hysterias ; the chief difference being that the anxiety hysteria has at its base a repression of ideas together with a certain amount of actual repression of emotions, whereas in the anxiety neurosis the repressed emotion is the chief factor, albeit repressed conflicting ideas are often to be discovered.

As regards neurasthenia I am myself rather doubtful as to its inclusion as a purely functional disease, and I shall give my reasons in a later paragraph. In the meantime it has so often a resemblance to and a mechanism consistent with these neuroses proper that rather for convenience sake than from conviction I have included it in this category.

1. Psycho-Neuroses (Hysterias)

These have as their basis repressed, unconscious ideas and conflicts which are of an unbearable nature to the individual, and which for some reason are in danger of becoming conscious. As we have shown in a previous chapter erotic energy may be repressed at two totally different stages: firstly, as regards the erotic impulse in early childhood; secondly, as regards the attainment of the erotic aim before, at or after puberty. In a suitable individual, if the repression begins to fail, if the sublimation be not good enough, and if some stimulus tends to bring to consciousness the repressed material (ideas, ideals, conflicts, etc.), a hysteria may result, and it does so as a further means of defence against the repression becoming conscious. It is, in other words, the last line of defence. The original repression may date from early childhood: a series of incidents in later life may add their energy to the tendency for repression to become conscious, but the power of repression may have been

sufficiently strong to keep the whole unconscious up to a certain period : the individual
during that period of his life may have remained
normal—in other words, the defence which
the censor of the mind exercised against the
repressed material has been adequate and successful. At last, however, some new conflict
may be so strong as to render further successful
defence impossible, unless the whole of the
repressed material which has been split off from
normal consciousness can obtain an outlet for
its energy in some manner still foreign to that
consciousness. What actually happens is that
such repressions do fail, the conflict tends
to become conscious, an attempt is made to
split it off from consciousness and to divert it
into another channel, and hysteria results—a
defence more or less successful in preventing
the unbearable ideas coming into normal consciousness. The particular form the hysteria
will take is determined by the prevailing idea
in the ensuing conflict between the censor and
the unconscious.

a. *Conversion Hysterias.*—The conflict in a
conversion hysteria is generally between a
repressed idea (wish) and an inhibition. The
inhibition may be internal, such as another idea
incompatible with the first one, or external
enforced by environment and circumstance.

The name arises because there is a *conversion* (with a splitting of consciousness) of the unpleasant idea from the mental to the physical plane. Let us take a hypothetical example : we will suppose an individual to have repressed successfully a mental conflict with its many added stimuli until a " last straw " is added which would normally bring the whole unbearable idea into consciousness. Let us further suppose that that individual is in the habit of using a phrase in very common use such as, " I feel awfully sick about it," referring of course not to physical sickness, but to an attitude of mind. The unbearable idea is about to become conscious, and the phrase, too, may be " on the tip of his tongue." The result is that a further temporary repression from consciousness takes place, and the individual turns the whole of his mental energy, which is making him " awfully sick " mentally into the physical plane, which makes him " awfully sick " physically. He actually begins to vomit upon the slightest provocation—has, in fact, acquired hysterical vomiting, and has also succeeded once more by means of this conversion in defending his conscious mind against the underlying unbearable ideas of the unconscious.

To quote a case of Brill's :—" A married woman of forty-nine years who suffered from hysteria for more than twenty-two years showed as one of her symptoms a very painful contracted and paralyzed right arm which had been so for more than three years. The muscles of the arm and shoulder region were completely anæsthetic and deep needle pricks were not perceived, but the slightest attempt to straighten out the member was most painful. Indeed the pain was the chief symptom. It would be impossible for me to give here the full analysis of the condition. I will merely mention some of the psychic constellations. Due to a number of sexual traumas sustained in childhood all sexual feelings were repressed and, as a result, she was totally frigid when she was married. Indeed coitus was both painful and disgusting to her. This produced marked marital unhappiness. Her husband failed to understand her condition, and what made matters worse was the fact that he found her masturbating in her sleep. When he first noticed it he was very indignant and tried to call her to account for it, but she continued to sleep; he tried to arouse her but she did not respond. He thought at first she was shamming, but finally concluded that ' she had a fit ' and reported the matter to the family physician. This somnambulistic state during which she masturbated was repeated on an average of five to six times a week. There was complete amnesia for this action. She at first refused to believe it, but she was finally convinced of it by her own sister, who saw her do it on the occasion of sleeping with her. She then sought the aid of a physician who gave her large doses of bromide and advised her to wear a sock over her hand and firmly tie her hand in complete flexion. While she was being treated for her masturbation it was reported to her that her husband carried on some illicit relations with one of the girls she employed. She absolutely refused to believe this, and no amount of urging on the part of her husband's own relatives could induce her to dismiss this girl. The latter was the daughter of a very poor woman, and it was out of compassion that she had taken her into her millinery establishment and taught her the business. This state of affairs continued for months. She was extremely jealous, yet her pride would not allow her to take any action in the matter. It was after a quarrel about some other matters, during which her husband grasped her by the right arm that it became painful and developed into the condition noted above. As she was the moving spirit in the millinery establishment the business had to be given up and she was totally incapacitated by her malady.

Here we see the conflict between the energy of desire and the repression. The repressed feelings made her consciously frigid and unconsciously passionate. When her masturbation was brought to her consciousness she took all the precautions to prevent it, but as usual she was unsuccessful. Her husband's faithlessness gave rise to another conflict. Her pride got the upper hand and she absolutely refused to believe what everyone else saw and what she herself could not fail to see. When her husband grasped her by this arm which was the cause of so much mental pain—it was the one with which she masturbated—the conversion took place. The symptom, as Freud puts it, was the result of a compromise between the opposing affects, one of which strove to bring to a realisation a partial impulse or a component of the sexual constitution, while the other strove to repress the same. This symptom, as we see, served a double purpose. It stopped the masturbation and incapacitated her to such an extent that her business had to be given up, and the girl who caused her so many pangs had to go. The pain was also the punishment for the underlying sexual desire. She never masturbated with her left hand, nor has she ever been seen masturbating since she was cured by psycho-analysis."

A very similar case came under my own

observation, which on account of its similarity, shows how often *we may expect* a given substratum of material in any patient, even at a superficial examination and before analysis takes place. The patient was a woman of about twenty-eight, and her trouble also was a paralysed right arm which was contracted with the elbow flexed at right angles—the hand and fingers also flexed and contracted. The patient from childhood upwards had lived in an atmosphere of religion of an extremely bigoted and dogmatic type. She had been brought up in almost entire ignorance of sexual matters, and with the idea that every thought, however remote, pertaining thereto, should be rigorously excluded from the mind. As a result of this she learned to look upon marriage itself as a mere cloak for making sin respectable, and to be avoided by anyone who wished to live the highest type of life. Nevertheless amazing as it may sound, she had from childhood upwards constantly practised masturbation, but without realising that this action had any gross sexual import, so profound was her ignorance of all sexual matters. A short period before her trouble with the arm commenced she read a book written by some well meaning, but ignorant person which had the object of opening people's eyes to the " dangers " of masturbation. In this book were the usual false statements which so often do harm, to the effect that masturbators become insane, get " softening " of the spinal cord, etc.   The patient realised with complete suddenness that she had been committing a perverted and bestial act of the worst kind and sustained the added shock that firstly her body and brain would shortly begin to suffer, and that secondly her immortal soul would be damned for ever.   The first conflict that arose was with her own habit.   This had grown upon her, and no amount of fear could subdue her desires in this direction.   For a short time the continuous thinking upon the subject, by auto-suggestion, and the unconscious counterwill increased her habit tenfold.   Then for a period she repressed the thoughts altogether and succeeded in overcoming her habit.   Then some stimulus caused the mental conflict to be about to become conscious once more ;   other repressed conflicts of an infantile nature, which I need not go into here, were also present ;   and suddenly she sought refuge in a conversion hysteria and gained *complete peace of mind* and apparently total forgetfulness at the expense of a paralyzed arm.   Analysis showed a very striking series of wish fulfilments similar to those observed in dreams.   Moreover, as the analysis proceeded, we found that as in dreams the one symptom was the disguise or symbol of several ideas requiring simultaneous expression. In the first place the paralysed arm was a punishment from God, and since she was being punished now she would avoid punishment hereafter. Secondly, it represented the physical effect of her evil doing, and since the harm done had resulted in a paralysed arm her spinal cord and brain would be safe from further trouble. Thirdly, the hand which had performed the deed was no longer able to do so, and hence desires were futile, hence also desires did not arise! Illogical reasoning no doubt, but quite good enough to form a path of safety for the unhappy mind of the patient, who, it must be remembered, was entirely unconscious of the cause of her trouble, or of the reasoning which had taken place in her unconscious. Under analysis the repressed material of course became conscious, some of the energy was sublimated, and readjustment of outlook and re-education in habits of thought, together with complete restoration of use of the arm, transformed her into a happy and useful woman once more.

Of course masturbation complexes are not behind all conversion hysterias. Those I have quoted hitherto merely happened to have this complex, and I am including them because of their simplicity and for purposes of comparison, as suggested above. Nearly every possible type of infantile repression with its ensuing conflict is represented in these conversion hysterias. A case is given by Freud in which a patient, a woman, had a very severe neuralgia of the facial nerve. Analysis showed that this represented physically the mental idea of a slap in the face, and was traced to an occasion upon which the husband had insulted the patient. I have not gone into the repressed infantile material in this case, as it is not necessary for our purpose here. One notices the similarity between the dream and the hysteria, *i.e.*, the production of a symbol or cartoon to express the repressed idea in a hidden form. This same patient of Freud's later exhibited the condition known as " globus hystericus." It represented " I cannot swallow that."

Conversion hysterias may have almost any physical sign or symptom, imitating with considerable accuracy almost any kind of actual lesion. Such symptoms may include practically any motor or sensory innervations or inhibitions; common forms met with are aphonias, paralyses contractures, anæsthesias, hyperæsthesias, pains, (especially neuralgias and abdominal pains), vomiting, diarrhœa, constipation, etc.

The Anxiety Hysterias.—These have a similar

mechanism to the conversion hysterias, but instead of the repressed complexes being converted into physical symptoms they disguise themselves on a second mental plane as either hysterical daydreams or phobias or " hysterical attacks." They differ from the conversion hysterias, however, in that the patients suffering from the latter as a rule are calm and happy, whereas those suffering from an anxiety hysteria frequently show signs of anxiety and apprehension, together with many of the signs and symptoms to be described under the anxiety neuroses. For the moment, however, we will confine ourselves to the formation of the phobias, hysterical daydreams, or hysterical " attacks."

Another point of difference between the anxiety hysterias and conversion hysterias is that in the anxiety hysterias there is nearly always some actual disturbance and abnormal repression of the sexual actions themselves with their attendant emotions. These specific sexual disturbances will also be discussed under the anxiety neuroses, for many of which they are directly responsible. In fact, one may say that in the anxiety hysterias the hysterical daydreams and phobias correspond with the repression of unpleasant conflicts, while the anxiety and physical signs correspond with the actual sexual disturbance.

A hysterical daydream or phantasy generally occurs in patients who have overcome masturbation and have got no other relief for an overstimulated sexual impulse, their powers of sublimation being undeveloped, *i.e.*, it is a conflict between a repressed wish and an internal inhibition. These hysterical daydreams generally show three distinct stages corresponding to the three stages in masturbation, in fact they may be looked upon as substitutes. The first stage is phantastic euphoria ; the the second stage is self absorption, when the patient withdraws from reality and is exalted and finds gratification in his secret thoughts ; the third stage is one of depression, corresponding closely with that depression found to follow the masturbatory act.

I cannot do better than quote in this connection one or two cases from Stoddart's New Psychiatry :

" 1.—A young woman used to imagine herself married to a handsome wealthy man. She had three most beautiful children ; they all lived in blissful happiness on a magnificent yacht and entertained most charming people. Then the whole structure crumbled ; her husband and children died and she was left alone in a terrible depression lasting for days.

2. A young weaver who thought he was

persecuted by his employer used to think what he would do if he had £400 a year. He imagined himself starting a shop and earning much money by oppressing his employees. His business grew until he had hundreds of people working for him. He became greater and greater until he found he had lost all his money on the Stock Exchange.

3. A young journalist imagines himself running a race and winning, when he is struck in the thigh by the spiked shoe of one of the competitors. He is bleeding and his trainers try to stop him, but he strikes them aside and runs on, winning the race. Then he collapses exhausted and is carried off amidst the cheers of the crowd.

4. A case from Freud : A lady imagined herself in delicate relationship with a piano virtuoso whom she did not know personally. In her fantasy she bore him a child. He deserted her, leaving her and her child in misery. She then suddenly found herself in tears in the street along which she happened to be walking.

Those who are familiar with psycho-analysis will discern the sexual complexes underlying these daydreams :—The desire for marriage in the first and last, the sadistic complex in the second, and the exhibition tendency in the third."

If the anxiety hysteria does not take the form of a daydream such as those given above it may appear as a phobia, but these phobias do not have a masturbatory complex behind them as a rule.

All phobias do not belong to the anxiety hysterias. Some are present in the compulsion hysterias (compulsion neuroses).

The phobias have been classified by Freud in the first instance, but his classification has been repeatedly modified as the result of new work, so that one cannot lay down a definite rule placing every particular phobia as a symptom of a particular neurosis. Originally phobias were divided into two groups :—The substituted and the unsubstituted phobias. The substituted phobias were those in which the phobia was of a similar nature to a conversion hysteria—that is, there was a definite substitution and outlet for definite repressed ideas and conflicts, the difference being that here we had substitution on a mental plane, whereas in the conversions hysterias the substitution took place in the physical plane. Such phobias were generally of a fairly definite nature, such as fear of cats, of needles or pins, of blood, etc., there being no limit to the variety of these fears, the chief point about them being that they were by no means vague, but strongly defined.

Unsubstituted phobias, on the other hand, were those which were not reducible to repressed ideas, but were apparently mere expressions of anxiety seizing upon a convenient experience. These belonged to the anxiety neuroses: examples of this type are claustrophobia, agoraphobia, the fear of thunderstorms and similar fears of a vague type. This classification as it stands, no longer holds good.

The anxiety hysterias certainly claim many substituted phobias which originally were classed with the compulsion neuroses. The so-called unsubstituted phobias are certainly sometimes to be classified amongst substituted phobias: for instance, I have found agoraphobia as a definite expression of a strongly repressed exhibitionism in which the phobia was an exaggerated reversal of the repressed desire. Agoraphobia represented the patient's idea of being too much exposed. Claustrophobia, on the other hand, has certainly appeared in one instance to be associated with a strongly marked Oedipus complex.

Thus although the classification has some foundation in fact we cannot yet state definitely which of the phobias indicates at once a particular hysteria or neurosis. It may, however, be taken that a person suffering from a phobia has either a compulsion neurosis or an anxiety hysteria, and the differential diagnosis between the two can easily be made when the physician goes further into the patient's history and condition.

Ernest Jones gives a good example of the material out of which a phobia may be built. Shortly, the case he describes is as follows : " A young man when standing on any height was afflicted with slight morbid anxiety nervousness, dread, giddiness, palpitation, sweating, etc., with a definite fear of jumping over the edge. This was always more severe when the edge overlooked deep water. The presence of any other man at the time made him afraid that the latter would throw him over : this fear did not apply to women. Association gave the following details : At the age of ten in a crowded concert hall an adult made him sit on the window ledge six feet above the stairs : he was very afraid of falling and in about half an hour got the friend to lift him down. (This incident, however, does not contain sufficient psychic damage in itself to cause the phobia, but it is evidently well adapted to bring the phobia into prominent evidence). The previous year his father had taken him up a tower 200 feet high, with a projecting balcony at the top. He was very greatly afraid of this balcony, although it was protected by railings, but his father laughingly forced him to walk round it, which he did in great terror. At the age of seven, a school teacher, a young man, had suspended him for a practical joke, upside down over a high wall, playfully threatening to let him drop, which also caused him great terror. At the age of three, a visitor picked him up in anger on one occasion and held him over a high water tank, into which he threatened to drop him. None of these facts, however, are sufficient to account for the phobia in themselves. In normal people such psychic traumata, and even more severe ones, often occur without leading to lasting phobias. Therefore it is plain that some other factor must be operative in cases where they do.

" Through the analyses of Freud and others it has been shown that a repressed wish is symbolised in the phobia, and that the continued action of this wish is responsible for the persistence of the phobia. Shortly, every phobia represents a compromise between one or more repressed wishes and the inhibiting forces that have repressed them. The activity of these wishes constitutes the essential and specific cause of the morbid mental state."

In discussing this phobia further Ernest Jones continues as follows : " The same phobia by no means always represents the same repressed

wish, though it does some wishes so much more
frequently than others that these may be called
types. The common types of wish that underlie the present phobia are the two following :
(1). The repressed desire to experience some
moral fall. This is symbolised by the physical
act of falling, in just the same way that the
spiritual idea of purification from sin is symbolised
in the material act of ablution with water
(baptism). The word ' fall ' is very commonly
employed to indicate the idea in question—
one need only mention such expressions as ' to
fall from grace,' ' fallen women,' ' backsliding
after conversion,' etc.—and the two connotations
of the word, the literal and the metaphorical,
generally become associated in the unconscious,
as do the various connotations of any given
word or of any pair of similarly sounding words
(2).—The repressed desire to make someone
else fall, either literally, (to throw them down
and hurt or kill them) or metaphorically (to
encompass their ruin). The present case is an
interesting example of the way in which this
cruel wish may become associated with, and
replaced in consciousness by, the fear of heights.
The chief mechanism involved is that of ' projection,' so common in both the disordered and
the normal (especially the infantile) mind. We
find it typically in the guilty conscience, for

instance in the fear of punishment for sin, and
a similar theme is to be met with in countless
dramas and novels in which the doom that the
villain prepares for the hero recoils on himself."
A murderously inclined man is afraid of being
murdered—he ascribes to others the evil desires
of his own heart : A liar does not trust an honest
man (Bernard Shaw justly says that the chief
punishment of a liar is not at all that he is not
believed, but that he cannot believe others) :
and so on.   In insanity one finds regularly that
delusions of persecution on the part of others
are the reflections, or projections, of evil thoughts
deep in the patient's own mind.   The whole
attitude of jealousy and fear of the rising
generation so frequent in older people (wonderfully dramatised in Ibsen's " Master Builder)
is partly due to a projection on to the former
of the hostile attitude that they themselves
when young indulged in towards their elders,
and now feel towards their juniors.   Instances
could be indefinitely multiplied, but these few
will probably serve to recall to the reader a
familiar human tendency.

The full analysis of the case described above
cannot be here related, but some of the principal
findings in the present connection were these.
As a baby the patient had been very sickly and
ailing ; his mother was of an unusually affec-

tionate disposition ; he was the only child : for these reasons he was unduly pampered by his mother, who doted on her first-born and nursed him night and day. He no doubt highly appreciated this affection, for when another child arrived—late in his second year—he showed every sign of resentment at this apparently superfluous intrusion into the circle of love where he had hitherto reigned supreme. Particularly did he object to renouncing the pleasure of being cradled in his mother's arms, which till now had always been open to him,* and the having to wait disconsolately while the baby was being nursed. The following trivial incident will illustrate this : One day when he was a little over two years old he called out vehemently to his mother, " Put the baby down in the cradle to cry, and *nurse me*."† The words " to cry " are especially to be noticed, these clearly being an unnecessary refinement of unkindness. No doubt his real feelings, the free manifestations of which were already being hampered by growing inhibitions, would have been more truly expressed in some such phrase

---

* It should not be forgotten that the height of a mother's arms is greatly magnified in the imagination of a little child, just as the size of any grown-up person is: hence the giants of mythology.

† The wording is in all probability correct, for the incident, which was often repeated as a family story, was told by the mother, who remembered it, as well as many others, very distinctly.

as, " Heave the little brat on to the floor, throw it away for good."

Another feature of importance was that throughout his childhood he had suffered greatly from fear of his father, as well as of the visitor mentioned above, a man who was closely identified in his mind with his father. Most of this fear was caused by a projection of the hostile thoughts bred by his jealousy of his father. He secretly hated his father, and nursed phantasies of killing him, so he ascribed to his father a similar hostility and also feared the latter's retribution if his evil thoughts became known. Therefore, when first the visitor, and later on the father, forced him into a situation where he was in peril of falling from a height (the tank and the tower incidents) his instinctive re-action was, " It's come at last. The all-knowing father has discovered my sinful thoughts, and he is going to do to me what I wanted to do to my little sister and to him."

The hate, jealousy and hostility that had arisen in earliest childhood had persisted in the patient's unconscious up to the present, in reference both to the relatives first concerned and other associated persons, on to whom it had later been transferred. Being of course repressed through the influence of moral training, and covered as well by a real love, it had never been consciously experienced in its full intensity, manifesting itself chiefly through endless friction and irritability, with occasional quarrels. The suffering and unhappiness resulting from these constituted one of the punishments that the patient's guilty conscience brought upon him for his cruel wishes. The phobia was another, a more direct self-punishment. When the pent-up wishes were released by being admitted to consciousness, and thereby weakened through the influence of various mental processes to which they had previously been inaccessible, a considerable improvement took place in his general mental condition, and the phobia became reduced to more normal proportions : the fires that had fed it being extinguished, there was nothing to keep it alive.

On the basis of this explanation it is intelligible that the most prominent part of the phobia had been the patient's fear that some other man would throw him over : in his unconscious his avenging father was always with him. The fear that he might himself jump over was a more direct expression of the repressed desire to do wrong, to " fall." The localisation to the neighbourhood of water was produced by a number of thoughts relating to the associations " throwing   down—killing—death— birth " that need not here be detailed.

According to the second of the two views discussed above, therefore, a phobia is a reaction to a repressed wish. It expresses the patient's fear (an emotion derived from the fear instinct) of a dissociated part of his own mind, of a dangerous tendency that he is afraid might overpower his better self : in popular phraseology it is " a fear of himself." The influence of any psychical trauma is merely incidental : it may be made use of by the phobia-building agency, thus, as in the present case, helping to determine the precise form this process shall take.

To avoid any possible misapprehension, I will repeat in conclusion two remarks already made above : first, that the particular repressed wish we have discussed is far from being the only one that may underlie a phobia of falling (nor was it by any means the only one in this case, though it was the chief one) ; and secondly, that the object of the present communication is not so much to produce any convincing evidence as to illustrate the contrast between two views by reference to a given case."*

* *Psycho-Analysis.* Ernest Jones.

CHAPTER X

The Functional Diseases (continued).

Compulsion Hysterias. (*Compulsion Neuroses*). The conflict in a compulsion hysteria is generally between a repressed wish and repressing forces which are not true inhibitions, and the condition always reveals a purely erotic basis, the symptoms actually being a substitution for repressed infantile erotic ideas and impulses. It thus differs slightly from the conversion hysteria in its primitive origin. We find also that in the compulsion hysteria the primitive repressed erotic wish is usually of the aggressive type, while in the conversion hysteria the repressed conflict is of sexual passivity. If we recover the early memories of a patient suffering from a compulsion neurosis, we shall probably find he was the aggressor in some form of erotic action or wish in infancy, whereas the patient suffering from a conversion hysteria or anxiety hysteria has been the one aggressed in infancy, he having played the passive role.

In the compulsion neuroses the actual mechanism of formation is much the same as in the conversion hysteria. There are strong repressions which are in danger of breaking down, and the energy of the repressed conflicts has turned into the neurosis as a safeguard against this and against this material becoming conscious. Instead, however, of the hysteria manifesting itself on the physical plane it manifests itself on another psychic plane, in the form of obsessions, doubts or irresistible ideas. The patient is thus *compelled* to act or to think in some manner which is disturbing to his conscious mind : he cannot help it. In some cases of compulsion hysteria phobias appear to be present, but it is possible that they really relate to a simultaneous anxiety hysteria. Moreover the obsessions on the psychic plane may manifest themselves as visual or auditory hallucinations. These are not, however, as a rule, delusions, at any rate in the early stages : for the patient may be quite aware of the fact that the voices he hears or the imaginary things which he sees are not real, although they may disturb him almost as much as if they were real : thus the compulsion neurosis differs from paranoid hysteria, where the patient has true delusions and really believes in the voices he hears speaking to him. It is by no means certain however, that a compulsion neurosis, if it become fixed and grow worse, may not

finally end in the patient having true delusions :
I have not yet been able to gather sufficient
evidence on this point to satisfy myself that it is
so. The obsessions of a patient suffering from
a compulsion neurosis are many and varied :
a large number of people have these in a mild
degree. For instance, a person is obliged to
step on the cracks of every third pavingstone,
or to count and to touch every tenth paling by
the roadside. A variation of this is found
when the patient is obliged to count everything
he sees. I had a patient who felt compelled
to stand momentarily upon all the manholes in
the pavement, and he found it impossible to
break the obsession himself.

Another form of compulsion neurosis is one
in which the patient feels bound to question
everything which comes under his notice :
to ask himself the most ridiculous questions,
such as whether the kettle on the hob is real,
or whether his wife's boots fit her. Everything
throughout the day, whether physical or intel¦
lectual, is met by a question on his part, not of
course expressed verbally, but a question asked
of himself, and a great worry because he is not
satisfied with the answer he gives himself. A
variety of this is met with in the fairly common neurosis known as *folie du doute*, in which
the patient cannot make up his mind about

anything. At the present moment I have a patient whom I am analysing, who until recently could not make up his mind in the morning which sock he would put on first, and throughout the day he was in a continual state of doubt about every trivial thing, and consequently got nothing done. On one occasion, he spent nearly two hours in the morning trying to make up his mind whether he should go to the pit or take other seats in a theatre for that night. The problem was so difficult that in the end he did not make up his mind at all. This form of compulsion neurosis is a fairly common one, and invariably one finds amongst other complexes present a strong Oedipus Complex, a homosexual complex, an anal-erotic complex, and an exhibitionist complex. A patient I recently analysed who had *folie du doute* gave on analysis a history of constipation as a child, with enemas administered per rectum by his mother : he showed in his dress and mannerisms strong exhibitionist tendencies ; he confessed to strong homosexual tendencies as a boy, which he stated had passed away, and that he was never attracted by women : finally, an attack of piles was associated in his mind with the first onset of his trouble. The attack of piles apparently acted as a stimulant to his anal-erotic complex, and especially his rectal examination by a doctor, his endeavours to prevent an operation by the daily anointing of the part with ointment, and the repetition of the use of an enema, which brought back to his mind the enemas administered to him by his mother somewhere about the age of four. It was obvious that he had a strong erotic fixation on his mother which was associated with anal-eroticism owing to his infantile experiences. This also accounted to some extent for his repressed homosexuality, in that he reverenced all women with the exaggerated reverence which he gave to his mother.

Another case of *folie du doute* which I have recently analysed, curiously enough came on immediately after the patient had had an operation for hæmorrhoids. Here again we had an anal-erotic history of a very definite kind dating right back to infancy. Here again the patient had strong exhibition tendencies, which not only manifested themselves in his dreams but also in the profession of his choice, which was that of a public speaker, with the alternative that he might, he stated, become an actor.

Other forms which the compulsion neurosis may take are those of pyromania, where the patient is unable to resist playing with fire, and may even end by being committed to prison for arson, though he is really no more to blame than a person suffering from acute appendicitis :

or kleptomania, also an unfortunate form of compulsion neurosis, and like the mania for collecting or for excessive tidiness, which it really resembles, often has as its basis a strong anal-erotic complex. If the kleptomaniac were analysed instead of being sent to prison, there would be some chance of his reformation : but the committal to prison will never cure him, for his obsession is completely beyond the control of his conscious mind, just as much as the paralysed arm in a conversion hysteria. Alchoholism and drug-taking may in many cases, though not in all, be classed among the compulsion neuroses : they are obvious acts outside the patient's normal control, which are substitutes for infantile forms of erotic satisfaction. Automatic writing is another obsessive act : here the patient may be quite unaware of the things he is writing down until he reads them over afterwards. The analysis of such writings may moreover reveal very speedily the complex which lies at the root of the neurosis. Occasionally one may even get an obsession resembling a trance, in which the patient will go to bed, and, though conscious, find himself unable to move or to speak. Or again, a person may be obsessed with the idea that he has some particular disease and that he must go to bed and stay there. Sometimes he will be obsessed with the idea of going to bed without having any idea of disease, and may stay there for months. A common form of symptom present in a compulsion neurosis is psychosexual impotence towards a particular person or persons.*

To sum up—the obsessions obviously may be of an endless variety, but the treatment of all of them is the same—psychoanalysis. For where the conversion hysteria may sometimes be completely cured by hypnotism, it is very rarely that a compulsion neurosis can be similarly cured. Relief may be found while the patient is actually in the doctor's hands, but sooner or later the trouble is nearly certain to recur.

Paranoid Hysteria.—Paranoid hysteria may possibly be regarded as the early stage in the formation of true paranoia. The mechanism and formation is much the same as regards repression and the side-tracking of the energy of unbearable ideas as we find in the conversion and the compulsion hysterias. It differs, however, very markedly in one respect, and that is in the phenomenon known as *projection*. The patient suffering from paranoid hysteria sees no defect

* A different type of psychosexual impotence is present in the Anxiety Neurosis

in himself, and realises no obsession nor physical ailment : he does, however, see imaginary defects in other people : in other words, his obsessions are *projected*. As in a compulsion hysteria he very likely will have auditory and visual hallucinations, but in paranoid hysteria he has true delusions and really believes in the voices he hears and in the demons which his mind conjures up : the auditory delusions are, however, much more common than the visual ones. The most striking point in paranoid hysteria is the patient's delusions concerning other people. He may have delusions of persecution, of amorousness, of jealousy or of exaltation, and if these delusions become strong enough the patient may merge into true paranoia and is likely to have homicidal tendencies towards the persons involved in his imagination. In all the cases of paranoid hysteria which I have seen repressed homosexuality seems to be the most striking feature : homosexuality is always very strongly developed in these subjects, although the patient may be totally unaware of it. The mechanism by which he projects his delusions has been summed up by Stoddart as follows :

"Unconsciously the paranoic always starts with the premise, " I love the man," (I am assuming the patient to be a male). The arguments in the several varieties of paranoia then run as follows :

Persecuted Paranoia.—" I love the man," an intolerable idea, therefore becoming " I do not love him ; I hate him." This by projection becomes, " He hates me. I am persecuted by him."

Exalted Paranoia.—" I love him," again an intolerable idea, therefore, " I do not love him, I love myself." This by projection becomes, " Everybody loves me." " I am a great person."

Religious Paranoia.—" I love him," being intolerable, becomes " I love Him " (spelt with a capital H), meaning " I love God." This by projection becomes, " God loves me." " I am the chosen one of God."

Amorous Paranoia.—The intolerable, " I love him," becomes " I do not love him, I love her." This by projection becomes, " She loves me."

Jealous Paranoia.—" I love him," as usual, is replaced by " I do not love him ; *she* loves him."

The mechanism of hypochondriacal paranoia is similar to that of exalted paranoia, " I love myself," becoming " I must take care of myself," and queralant (*sic*) paranoia is only a special variety of persecuted paranoia."

It seems as if many cases of paranoia if analysed

at a sufficiently early stage might be cured, instead of ending as they so often do in a lunatic asylum : and according to accounts given by Ferenczi and others even cases which are far advanced appear to be curable. Certainly the cases I have analysed have all been very early ones, and out of about half a dozen I have only had one relapse. In that particular case the patient was so averse from analysis and from me that although he had improved for a time we could not go on with the work, and he is now in an asylum, having attempted among other things to burn down his father's house.

One must lay particular stress on the fact, however, that all paranoid cases are not, with our present knowledge, suitable for treatment. I am particularly careful in selecting cases for treatment, not only because some are very resistant to treatment (for you will remember that paranoid hysterias do not as a rule admit that there is anything the matter with them), but also because they have a habit of projecting such ideas as persecution upon the physician, who is then liable to run a distinct danger from his patient. · One cannot emphasise too strongly the necessity for very careful discrimination in selecting a paranoid patient for treatment. There are, however, cases of compulsion hysteria that very closely resemble and are often mistaken for paranoia : these are all amenable to, and excellent cases for, psychoanalysis.

Dementia Proecox.—A similar mechanism is stated to be present in dementia praecox, with a reversal of the procedure. Instead of projecting his ego upon the world—the patient withdraws everything into his innermost self. I have, however, not yet attempted to analyse a case of this kind, nor have I been satisfied that any of the cases that have been reported to me as being cases of dementia praecox have in fact been such. I therefore include this disease in this chapter with some misgiving, and more because several well-known analyists abroad have vouched for it than because I am as yet convinced.

ᴇ *Anxiety Neuroses.*—As stated earlier, the anxiety neuroses have as their basis a repression of psychic energy rather than of conflicting ideas or wishes, although of course in no case can we quite separate the energy underlying the emotion from some accompanying idea. Here there arises the difficulty in separating the anxiety neurosis from the anxiety hysteria, and whether we are to call the manifestations the one or the other depends largely upon the number of repressed complexes present as opposed to the amount of accumulated emotion. Thus the anxiety neurosis is very often accompanied by a phobia, especially of the so-called unsub-stituted type. The mechanism of the anxiety neurosis seems to consist in the gradual accumu-lation or repression of psychic energy : this remains unused and finding no outlet, in its endeavour to escape from repression causes many physical and mental manifestations of a widely differing type. The mental manifestations are chiefly those of anxiety in various forms, and the tension caused by this mental anxiety appears to react physically, even appears to produce such symptoms as changes in the secretory glands. We may liken the mind of the person suffering from an anxiety neurosis to a steam boiler with the safety valve closed down : when the steam pressure continues to rise but finds no outlet it finally bursts the joints between the plates and breaks out through the rivet holes and other places.° So the anxiety neurosis appears to be a kind of leaking or bursting out of psychic energy in the wrong direction. ° The continued repression of normal psychic energy appears to be able to cause this neurosis in normal life : the chief causes are those directly connected with sex, the three commonest causes being firstly, long engage-ments between men and women in which there is continuously erotic desire which is repressed with difficulty and never consummated. Secondly, coitus interruptus, by which we mean that type of coitus where the man in order to avoid adding to his family makes a regular habit of withdrawing himself from his wife before the actual emission takes place. In this case the emotional discharge is far from normal and is quite inadequate to the occasion. A gradual accumulation of psychic energy seems to take place, which at a suitable moment manifests itself as an anxiety neurosis. Thirdly, we have coitus reservatus. In this case either the man or the woman deliberately and habitually holds back his emotional discharge for several minutes, so that it may take place simultaneously with the emotional discharge of the other person, who takes a longer period to reach that final stage of coitus. But these emotions are by no means the only ones which appear to cause the anxiety neurosis. The continued repression for long periods of fear or of disgust such as has been caused in many by the recent war, lead to a very similar condition, though the resulting anxiety neurosis has very often been termed " shell shock."

Characteristics of an Anxiety Neurosis.—In giving the signs and symptoms which may be present in this disease I must warn readers not to expect to meet all or even most of them in any one case. Often perhaps only one trivial symptom is complained of, and no physical signs at all may be present. In other cases, however, we may have very nearly the whole syndrome.

The Anxiety Neurosis shows all the signs and symptoms of anxiety, hence its name. We see it in a mild and temporary form in students about to undergo an examination, or runners about to commence a race. It is common knowledge that in these instances the muscles may be held tense. There is increased rapidity of both respiration and pulse. There may be a certain amount of sweating, and the desire for more frequent micturition is common. That is our temporary and trivial anxiety neurosis. In the major and chronic forms we have to tabulate, however, a much larger variety of symptoms and signs.

Symptoms.—The patient may complain of fits of depression, of great irritability of temper, of worrying about trifles, of impaired powers of concentration and memory, of lack of confidence, headaches, giddiness, and even actual collapse following this giddiness, in which he loses consciousness. He may term this collapse a " fit," but it is more probably due to a vasomotor change leading to an ordinary fainting attack. Insomnia is another common complaint. Sleep may be broken by terrible dreams, and in the case of the war neurosis particularly, by battle-dreams, which often repeat the patient's own experiences most vividly. He may further complain of morbid anxieties and fears, *i.e.*, the unsubstituted phobias of which we spoke previously, of disturbed appetite and feelings of nausea, but without any vomiting. He often complains also of frequency of micturition, especially at night, and of sexual impotence. He may state that he is disturbed by the slightest noise, that he is very readily excited, that on excitement he gets palpitation of the heart and shortness of breath. On excitement also he may be inclined to stammer, especially when meeting strangers. Occasionally he complains of anginal attacks, with a fear of impending death. Generally speaking, he lives in a state of apprehension which may be very mild or quite acute. The patient is very easily exhausted, probably because he is using so much energy in making himself in a tense condition generally.

Signs.—The patient looks anxious and worried. He may have general tremors of the body or localised tremors of the hands, fingers or tongue. His deep reflexes are exaggerated. He may on occasions have a spurious ankle clonus, or even rombergism. His muscles are commonly hypertonic, and he is unable to relax them. If his arm be lifted it does not fall instantly, even when he is told to allow it to do so. Just as the muscles are in a state of hypertension so do the arteries appear to be for his blood pressure is often 20mm. to 40mm. higher than the normal for his age and general condition.* There are other vaso-motor disturbances as evidenced by alterations of his secretions. He may sweat profusely from time to time or on the slightest exertion. Sometimes night sweats are complained of. His gastric secretions appear to be disturbed. The hands and feet may be cyanosed and cold. Among the muscles held in a rigid condition the diaphragm particularly may be mentioned. In many cases I have seen it appeared to be entirely without action. The breathing was entirely of the costal type and abdominal breathing could not be performed by the patient even with voluntary effort. In such cases the lower border of the lungs appeared to be drawn upwards so that the apex beat of the heart became more than usually visible. In connection with this even when there was a certain amount of diaphragmatic breathing a systolic murmur is often heard over the apex of the heart, but it is not conducted towards the axilla,

* "Relation of Blood Pressure to the Psychoneuroses," Paul Bousfield. "The Practitioner," November, 1918.

nor indeed in any direction. The explanation of this is difficult to give, as it is certainly not due to any lesion of the heart, but probably to a disturbed relation between the pericardium and its surroundings. Tachycardia and dyspnœa are very common. Diarrhœa or constipation may be present. The patient may be very emotional and weep during examination. Stammering is often present in those cases where the respiration is disturbed. If, however, it be present in those cases where the breathing is not disturbed, I generally find we are dealing with an hysterical symptom rather than with one due to the pure anxiety neurosis.

A few words on the treatment of anxiety neurosis will not be out of place here. Analysis may or may not be required, according to the amount of contemporaneous anxiety hysteria present. It will, however, be obvious from our statement of the causes of the anxiety neuroses that one of the essential things is for the patient to rectify as far as possible any abnormal sexual conditions, and for this purpose, of course, the requisite advice from the physician is necessary. This must often be supplemented, however, with a certain amount of psychoanalysis in order that the physician may discover the mental complexes which lie at the root of the patient's abnormal behaviour.

This particularly applies to those anxiety neuroses which have their origin in complexes concerned with the instinct of propagation.

In those connected with the instinct of self-preservation* (fear, etc.,) a rather different method of removing the repressed emotional energy may be used. In a typical case arising out of the war the patient has repressed the instincts of fear, disgust, etc., over a prolonged period, and although he is now no longer in physical danger we generally find that he is still very strenuously repressing his previous fears and all incidents connected with them. He refuses to discuss the war, and more particularly dislikes any reference of his own personal experiences. If he is asked *why* he will not discuss these with his friends, he will probably say that it thoroughly upsets him or makes him ill in different ways. Here we have to make use of what is known as " abreaction." The patient must be made to talk daily for at least half an hour, and preferably longer, of his own worst experiences. He must not try to avoid them, but to face them in every detail, and the fact must be pointed out to him that at the beginning he may be very emotional and upset by such conversations, and that this is, in fact, a good sign, for he is, so to speak, gradually allowing

*Erotic material is frequently to be found in these cases also.

the emotions natural to the situations which he is discussing to be worked off.

It will be found that these battle-dreams which are so common in occurence begin almost immediately to diminish in frequency as soon as the conversation upon his experiences has begun, and as a rule at the end of about three weeks they have almost entirely ceased. It is quite true that in some instances, at this period, the battle-dreams do not cease, but change somewhat in their character, and under these circumstances they probably refer to something other than his actual war experiences. In other words, his anxiety neurosis may have a considerable reference to other repressed emotions. Indeed, one frequently finds that there is a erotic as well as a war basis for the anxiety neurosis in question.

Other accessory treatment is often advisable in these neuroses. Concentration and memory exercises are of great assistance : exercises for the relaxation of muscles are also very valuable. I have pointed out that the breathing is often of costal character, and here exercises in abdominal respiration are of great value, not only in relieving the general condition, but also effecting an improvement in cases where stammering is a marked complaint.

In one or two instances I have found that no

amount of persuasion would induce a patient to use his diaphragm, and in these cases I have used adhesive strapping, and have strapped the patient's thorax and clavicles in the position of forced expiration. He is then obliged at once to use his diaphragm, and may be left in this condition for two or three days until the habit is established. Suggestion may be used for curing the insomnia and relieving the headache, and there are certain drugs which may also be used with advantage. I have analysed a good many of these anxiety neuroses of war, and in almost all instances have found an abnormal unconscious homo-sexual constituent, which has been stimulated by the patient's experiences.

I pointed out that a large number of these cases had a raised blood pressure, and small doses of nitro-glycerine given every night before retiring to bed serve to reduce this somewhat, and, by reducing it, to relieve the patient's headache and increase his possibilities of sleeping. In cases where the blood pressure is more than 40mm. above the normal, I generally find a history of recent constipation, with probable lower bowel infection causing auto-intoxication. I find a course of senna and vegetable charcoal of the greatest benefit in such cases in reducing the blood pressure. I follow this up with nitro-glycerine. For localised sweating of a pronounced character, a lotion containing a little belladonna is frequently of service, and if this be gradually reduced in strength it will often remain just as efficacious, as a large element of suggestion enters into the case once the patient has found the value of the lotion.

Neurasthenia.—As I have already stated, this is a much abused term. True neurasthenia is a comparatively rare complaint. It has a very definite syndrome of symptoms, and but few physical signs of a definite nature.

The actual causative factor of neurasthenia is by no means clear to me. I am not at all sure that it should be classed as a pure functional disease. Freud and other writers state that neurasthenia is always due to sexual excess, and more particularly to excessive masturbation. Personally, I doubt this fact. I have not found it by any means constantly at the foundation of cases I have gone into very thoroughly. Other writers are inclined to view neurasthenia as due to a definite auto-intoxication, either from the intestines or from disturbed secretions of the ductless glands. To my mind the ætiology is by no means sufficiently clear for us to be dogmatic, especially since two important physical factors are often found in conjunction with neurasthenia, namely, great loss of weight and a dilated stomach. Probably both schools of thought are correct. There may be more than one cause, or they may act in combination.

Characteristics of Neurasthenia.—The patient complains of excessive fatigue on any exertion, whether mental or physical, and after a time the mere thought of effort may exhaust the patient completely in advanced cases. He may have headaches, generally occipital, but more frequently he complains of a sense of pressure on the skull, particularly in the neighbourhood of the vertex. There may also be indefinite spinal pain or weakness, and a common complaint is of a peculiar " wriggling " sensation in the occipital region or over the cervical spine. Insomnia is another occasional complaint, but this is by no means frequent : in advanced cases the powers of memory and concentration are impaired, and there is loss of self confidence. On exertion the patient may break into a profuse perspiration.

Signs.—The muscles are generally flaccid : the deep reflexes are sluggish or even sometimes absent : the blood pressure is usually low for the patient's age and general condition. Too much attention should not, however, be paid to the deep reflexes or to the blood pressure, as the patient often has some other disturbing element in his condition : this may be either of a physical nature, or quite commonly he may have a superimposed anxiety neurosis. Marked general asthenia with loss of weight, amounting frequently to two or three stones is common. Very frequently the patient complains of flatulence and abdominal discomfort, and examination will show considerable dilatation of the stomach. The patient frequently has hypochondriacal ideas but he has no phobias nor obsessions. Indeed, the hypochondriacal ideas are not to be wondered at, since his loss of weight and gastric trouble together with his other symptoms are enough to suggest many diseases to any normal mind, especially if he passes through the hands of a physician who states that he can find nothing wrong with him.

It will be observed that neurasthenia has certain points in common with a mild anxiety neurosis, as also with many organic diseases such as chronic interstitial nephritis, glycosuria, malignant disease, and other debilitating lesions, and an extremely careful examination should, of course, be made before a diagnosis of neurasthenia is made.

Treatment.—With regard to treatment of neurasthenia all forms of psychotherapy give very unsatisfactory results. If there is a history of any excessive sexual action this must, of course, be remedied. A short analysis is often useful, because an anxiety hysteria is frequently present : moreover, a short analysis reveals the patient's likes and dislikes, and enables one to map out the right kind of occupation for the patient during treatment. In any case the analysis is of some benefit to the patient, for it invariably improves the mental balance and methods of utilising energy in any persons, however normal they may appear to be. The main treatment in neurasthenia should consist in rest, change of company and abode, regulated exercise and light but enjoyable employment. As a rule such treatment should occupy at least six months. I do not advocate the patient being sent to the sea-side, as this is often too stimulating : rather, I prefer a country village. In cases where there is any gastric disturbance, special importance should be attached to diet, and if necessary suitable drugs should be administered. The Weir Mitchell treatment also often gives excellent results if properly carried out.*

---

* "An Outline of Psychotherapy" Paul Bousfield, May, 1919, A lecture delivered before the Deputy Commissioners of Medical Service—reprinted Medical Press May 7th, 14th and 21st, 1919.

CHAPTER XI

TECHNIQUE OF PSYCHO-ANALYSIS

PSYCHO-ANALYSIS has as its object the following up of trains of ideas and thoughts from the conscious into the unconscious mind in such a manner that repressed complexes may be revealed and brought into full consciousness.

With a selected starting-point the patient must give free associations. By free associations we mean ideas which come into his mind when he fixes his attention on the starting-point— such ideas being entirely uncontrolled either by criticism or resistance on his part. Secondary ideas are again obtained from these first, and so on. As would be supposed, however, it is by no means easy for a patient to get rid of his own resistance and his tendency to criticise. For the purpose of demonstrating in some measure what we mean by free association, I will first describe shortly what is known as " Jung's Association Method."

I. THE ASSOCIATION METHOD.—This method is based upon the fact that for every stimulus we receive a suitable reaction is forthcoming; that should the stimulus touch upon some unpleasant or repressed material in our minds, we shall react in a different manner from that in which we should react were the stimulus to touch neutral or colourless material in our mind. For example, if a highly nervous woman saw a mouse on the floor she might instantly shriek and draw her feet up on to a chair; whereas if she saw a piece of paper on the floor she would do nothing of the kind. In the one case the stimulus touches a complex which is unpleasant and evokes an emotion, in the other no emotion is evoked.

In Jung's association method, instead of using a large number of actual situations in order to find out which of them will evoke emotion in a patient he tests them with a large number of words, among which are certain words which may stimulate nearly every possible emotion. A list of words, generally about one hundred is taken: a large number of them are quite commonplace and should not act in any way as an abnormal stimulus to anyone. Scattered through these, however, are carefully chosen words which are likely to touch upon one or some of the complexes of the patient and arouse the emotion which has been repressed in connection with that complex. Each word is read out slowly to the patient, who is instructed to give in reply the first word that comes into his head in association with the word read out. He is further informed that he must not criticise nor resist : that if the word that occurs to him is vulgar or apparently not strictly to the point it will make no difference—he must still say that word. Now these words act, though in a less powerful way, exactly as a similar situation would act, and they serve as stimuli to evoke repressed material in the mind. An innocuous word like " ink " would be readily answered by such a word as " pen," but to a patient who was terrified of mice the word " mouse " would call up a picture in which the mouse figured. Although of course the patient would not react absolutely in the same way as in the situation just described, nevertheless he would react in such a way that it would be noticeable either from his manner, or from some slight hesitation timeable in fractions of a second, or from some slight internal struggle which could be registered on a galvanometer. Thus in reading over this list of words each reply of the patient's is timed by a stop watch, reading in fifths of a second or in some other suitable manner. His bearing and manner are closely watched, and any faulty or unusual methods of answering are noted.

When the list has been read through once and his associations written down, as a general rule one repeats the process and asks the patient where possible to repeat the same word as before, but where not possible again to give the first word that comes into his head. It will often be found that a certain proportion of his associations are different on this second reading, and the stimulus words to which he reacts differently are noted, for these are important.

It might be thought that a critical —that is to him an unpleasant stimulus word— to which it took him several seconds to find an association would register itself more indelibly on his memory than a neutral word—a word that awakes no particular memories in his mind, but this is not the case. The inward perturbation, however slight, prevents him from fixing his attention on the association he gives, and as a rule it will be found that the stimulus words that are to him critical words, are the ones to which he fails to react twice in the same manner. So infallible is this method that by a physician who has practised it the repressed complexes of any normal person can be detected : however normal the person he cannot prevent his reactions to any critical stimuli which touch upon repressed conflicts. By this method criminals can be made to reveal their guilt : indeed, Jung gives an excellent example of this in his work on Analytical Psychology.

Now as to the more detailed work in Jung's method. The average reaction time found for the majority of persons is 2.4 seconds per word. In some cases one will find that the patient habitually takes very much longer to react to every word, whether it touch a complex or not. This shows that the patient finds difficulty in adapting himself to the physician— that a high degree of disturbance in adjustment is present, and that in a certain sense he is but imperfectly adapted to reality. Again we shall observe two chief ways in which patients react ; they may react with outer and sound associations rather than with inner associations, thus following lines of least resistance by reactions with easy speech combinations : in these patients there is a disturbance of attention producing this shallow reaction : or others may react with inner associations, and in these we may conclude there is concentration of the attention.

Again, many persons—especially those of a neurotic type, will react with more than one word : not satisfied with following out instructions, they give several words or explanatory sentences : they are unable to suppress the ideas which occur to them. By their desire to supplement they show a desire to give the physician more than he wants and make great efforts to find further associations so that a completely satisfactory answer may be given. Jung has shown that this signifies that such persons have a constant tendency to give others more feeling than is required or expected : while Freud has shown that this is a method of compensating for an inner want of satisfaction and voidness of feeling. It is one of the characteristics of many hysterical persons, who allow themselves to be carried away by everything, to attach themselves to everything, to promise much and to perform little. Another characteristic of this type of person is a tendency to take everything personally, and to defend himself as though against being misunderstood by careful explanation. Thus to the stimulus word " to pray " such a person, instead of replying by perhaps the one word " church," would say : " church ; God ; one should not pray for material things ! " or to such a word as " marry " he might reply : " wife ; husband ; children ; I am not thinking of being married."

Yet another point to be noticed, especially, in carrying out this method, is the repetition of certain stimulus words by the patient as if he did not quite understand or had not heard correctly. This arises from the same motive as that which induces him to give elaborate explanation of his reaction to the words that are for him critical : it means that he is treating the word as if it has some personal reference—as if it were a difficult personal question. It will often be found in going over the list of words that the patient reacts to many of them by using the same reaction word ; when this word recurs frequently it is sure to have some significance and is worth investigation. For instance, Jung quotes a case in which the patient repeated the word " short " a great many times, and often in places where it had no obvious connection. He could give no reason for this repetition. ɔ From experience Jung knew that such predicates always relate either to the test person himself or to one very near to him, and assumed that by this word " short " he designated himself and that it touched on an unpleasant complex. " The test person was of very small stature. He was the youngest of four brothers who in contrast to himself were all tall. . He was always the ' child ' of the family. He was nicknamed ' short ' and treated by all as the ' little one.' This resulted in a total loss of self-confidence. Although he was intelligent, and despite long study, he could not decide to present himself for examination, but finally became impotent and merged into a psychosis in which whenever he was alone he took delight in walking about in his room on his toes in order to appear taller. The word ' short ' therefore stood to him for a great many painful experiences. This is usually the case with these so-called ' perseverated ' words ; they always denote something of importance in the individual psychology of the test person.".

It often happens that so much emotion is evoked by one of the critical stimulus words that it is carried on to the next word or two, although these may be neutral, and we may find either that the reaction time for these neutral words is longer than would be expected, or on the second repetition a different reaction word may be reproduced to them as well as to the critical word that preceded them.

Jung divides individuals into three principal types as regards their reactions to his association method : firstly, *an objective type,* or those whose reactions are undisturbed ; secondly, *a complex type,* or those who show disturbance in the way mentioned above and which is caused by the stimulation of the repressed material of their complex or complexes ; thirdly, *a definition type,* or those who always give an explanation or definition of the stimulus word. For instance the third type would reply to the stimulus word " *tree,*" " fruit ; " to " *table,*" " a piece of household furniture ; " to " *promenade* " " an activity ; " to " *father* " " chief of the family." Such replies are generally found in stupid people, and are quite usual from imbeciles ; but they are also given by persons who are not stupid, but who do not wish to be taken for stupid ; the test person is of the opinion that it is an examination in intelligence and therefore he directs his attention to the significance of the stimulus word and by so doing makes his associations similar to those of an idiot. All idiots, however, do not react with definitions ; probably only those react in this way who have a secret wish to appear smarter than they are—*i.e.*, those to whom their very stupidity is painful. Jung calls this complex the " *intelligence complex.*" Persons with an intelligence complex are usually unnatural and constrained ; they wish to be more than they are, to exert more influence than they are able to. They use high-sounding quotations, their replies are stilted and contain foreign words and other intellectual ornaments, and this to impress others with their intelligence and to compensate for their own painful feeling of stupidity.

This definition type is closely allied to what Jung calls the *predicate type*, where personal judgment is expressed upon every stimulus word thus : *flower*, pretty ; *money*, convenient; *animal,* ugly; *knife,* dangerous; *death,* ghastly. In the definition type the *intellectual* significance of the stimulus word is prominent, in the predicate type its *emotional* significance.

Some predicate types show great exaggeration in their reactions such as: *pain,* horrible; *to sing,* heavenly; *mother,* ardently adored; *nice,* holy.

In the definition type we have pointed out that an intellectual make-up is simulated, and that it really conceals a lack of intelligence. In the predicate type the more emotional expression conceals or compensates for emotional deficiency. Jung shows this conclusion in a most interesting way in the following: " On investigating the influence of the familiar mileus on the association type it was found that young people seldom possess a predicate type, but that this type increases in frequency with advancing age. In women it increases a little after the fortieth year, in men after the sixtieth. This is the precise time when, owing to the deficiency of sexuality, there actually occurs considerable emotional loss. If a test person evinces a distinct predicate type it may be inferred that a marked internal deficiency is thereby compensated." One cannot, however, reason conversely that an inner emotional deficiency must produce

* These examples are taken from Jung's Analytical Psychology.

a predicate type. A predicate type can also betray itself through external behaviour, as, for example, through a particular affectation, or through enthusiastic exclamations and the constrained-sounding language so often observed in society."

With regard to the *complex type* there is in these a reference to our definition and predicate types, but while these show a positive tendency to exert a definite influence on the physician the complex type show a tendency to conceal the complex not only from the physician but from themselves as well.

The following is the list of words I generally use. They are largely based upon Jung's own list with alterations made where the translated word does not bear the same significance or has an awkward sound in the English language. Additional words are often interspersed when I have occasion to suspect the presence of any particular complex and wish to get confirmation of this from the patient :

1. head.	7. ship.
2. green.	8. to pay.
3. water.	9. window.
4. to sing.	10. friendly.
5. dead.	11. to cook.
6. long.	12. to ask.

13. cold.
14. stem.
15. to dance.
16. village.
17. late.
18. sick.
19. pride.
20. table.
21. ink.
22. angry.
23. needle.
24. to swim.
25. voyage.
26. blue.
27. lamp.
28. to sin.
29. bread.
30. rich.
31. tree.
32. to prick.
33. pity.
34. yellow.
35. mountain.
36. to die.
37. salt.
38. new.
39. custom.
40. to pray.
41. money.

42. foolish.
43. paper.
44. despise.
45. finger.
46. expensive.
47. bird.
48. to fall.
49. book.
50. unjust.
51. frog.
52. to part.
53. hunger.
54. white.
55. child.
56. to take care.
57. lead pencil.
58. sad.
59. plum.
60. to marry.
61. house.
62. dear.
63. glass.
64. to quarrel.
65. fur.
66. big.
67. carrot.
68. to paint.
69. part.
70. old.

71.	flower.	91.	to choose.
72.	to beat.	92.	hay.
73.	box.	93.	pure.
74.	wild.	94.	contented.
75.	family.	95.	ridicule.
76.	to wash.	96.	to sleep.
77.	cow.	97.	month.
78.	friend.	98.	nice.
79.	luck.	99.	woman.
80.	lie.	100.	to abuse.
81.	behaviour.	101.	red.
82.	narrow.	102.	to fight.
83.	brother.	103.	boy.
84.	to fear.	104.	dish.
85.	stork.	105.	to love.
86.	false.	106.	number.
87.	anxiety.	107.	girl.
88.	to kiss.	108.	tired.
89.	bride.	109.	ball.
90.	door.	110.	to tear.

2. GENERAL MANAGEMENT OF ANALYSIS.—
From the foregoing something will have been
gathered as to what is meant by free association,
which is the essential factor in psycho-analysis.
The physician does not, however, start at once
by asking the patient for free associations. It
is necessary first to establish some sort of rapport
between himself and his patient, and to ascertain
something about his conscious mind before en-

deavouring to bring up material from the unconscious. One first gets all the information possible about his symptoms : when they came on first, when there have been exacerbations, and when the patient has been more or less free from them. At the same time one asks him whether he can ascribe any of his symptoms to any definite happenings connected closely with them, and one ascertains as much as possible of the patient's occupation and environment at the onset of his illness and during exacerbations. This generally fills up the first visit to the patient, which occupies about an hour. On the next visit I get from the patient the critical dates in his life history, together with other facts : such as the respective ages of his parents, the dates upon which he went to various schools, became engaged to be married, was married, the date of the death of either of his parents, the number of brothers and sisters and their ages, the general history of his health throughout life and something of his early life and environment. In some cases, but by no means in all, I ask for something of the sexual history of the patient, of his earliest recollections of this, and any habits of body or of mind which he may have formed. Before referring to the sexual history, however, we must be careful to sum up the general attitude of the patient, for it is by no means the wisest thing to do, and in many instances it is better left to reveal itself bit by bit during the analysis. However, in cases where it is advisable to do this we may succeed in shortening the analysis somewhat, and in reducing the resistance of the patient to further revelations. In the case of well-educated and intelligent patients it is well to explain at this stage something of the nature of analysis and the constitution of the unconscious mind, and to point out what we mean by repressed conflicts and by infantile sexuality. At the same time it is essential to make it clear that we are not dealing with these matters from the point of view of right and wrong, but in the scientific spirit of an unbiassed investigation : and indeed, that we do not regard the patient as responsible for his repressed conflicts, but that they are the outcome of his early environment and education, which, of course, were outside his control. ₤ It is as well to point out at the same time that he is not alone in possessing displaced or repressed infantile forms of sexuality : that the same may be true of even normal people, and that the only difference between him and a normal person lies in the degree of repression on the one hand and the power of resistance, the amount of sublimation, etc., on the other. By having a general chat on these lines we shall put the patient much more at his ease, and diminish to some extent the resistance in yielding the superficial matter which will appear first.

Our next step is to begin the analysis proper. Personally, I very often begin with the word association test, not only because it gives an insight into some of the chief complexes, but because it introduces the patient in an easy manner to free association, and accustoms him to understanding what is meant by it. In carrying out the analysis one wishes the patient to forget as far as possible the presence of the physician : for this purpose he should be made to sit in a comfortable chair or to recline upon a couch so placed that, while the physician can watch the patient's face and manner, the latter cannot study the physician. It is also advisable that disturbing noises or other stimuli from without should be as far as possible excluded. The patient's attention is then directed to a word, as in the above-mentioned association method, or to the first onset of his neurosis, or to some habitual action of his, or indeed to almost anything that will serve as a starting-point, and he is asked to say whatever comes into his mind when he thinks of this, without prejudice, without criticism and without resist-ance. He is encouraged to talk and to take

his own line of thought, and must not be forced
by the physician into the particular path which
the latter thinks will lead to what is at the
basis of the neurosis. If he wanders too far
away from the point he may from time to time
be recalled to the starting-point, or his attention
may be directed to something he has associated
with it and further associations may be asked
for, but care should be taken that no hint is
given as to the inner meaning of any statements
the patient may make unless a point is reached
where he has given such overwhelming evidence
of what is present in his unconscious mind that
he cannot fail to recognise the truth of its
existence when it is put before him.

It must be remembered that psycho-analysis
has nothing to do with hypnotism nor suggestion,
and the beginner will often have a hard task
to prevent himself from giving suggestions to
the patient which he thinks will hurry on the
analysis since to him certain complexes, repressions or fixations have become abundantly
clear. It must be remembered that as a rule
the analysis cannot be hurried: it must be
allowed to take its course, except in rare instances, which the analyst will only recognise
after he has had considerable experience.

Now the royal road to the patient's
unconscious is by means of the analysis

of dreams, for, as we have already stated, dreams, amongst other things, fulfil the patient's repressed wishes in a disguised form. We therefore direct the patient after the first three or four sittings to remember his dreams as far as possible and to relate them on each occasion on which he visits us. If he says that he does not dream it is best to inform him that we probably all dream, but that some like himself do not remember their dreams upon awakening, and that if he goes to bed with the firm intention of remembering his dreams he will be sure to do so. This expedient will be found as a general rule to produce the right result. It is as well to ask the patient whether he remembers any vivid dreams which he used to have in childhood or which have recurred repeatedly, as this will convey much to the analyst, and will be useful for comparative purposes at a later stage. During the first half dozen visits or so I ask the patient to take a pencil and paper to bed with him and to write down his dreams as fully as possible, as it is as well to keep a record of these early dreams also for future reference. I do not, however, let him read these dreams out to me, but make him repeat them to me, while I preserve a written copy. One often asks the patient to repeat the dream twice, because there are often points of difference between the two versions: slight though they may be, these points of difference indicate points of strong resistance in the latent meaning of the dream, and to these the analysis should be especially directed.

One of the reasons why a beginner at analysis is often inclined to point out some unmistakable revelation of infantile sexuality in one of the patient's early dreams is that he is afraid the patient may not have another dream like this one, and that the opportunity which appears so suitable may not come again. It should be borne in mind, however, that any infantile material of this kind which has not become fully conscious to the patient is sure to reappear at different periods when that particular repressed conflict is stimulated, and that if it is of importance in the neurosis it will probably be stimulated pretty frequently. He may therefore with full assurance refrain from forcing his interpretation of the dream upon the unconscious patient, with the knowledge that when the right time comes he will have several dreams in further corroboration of what was evident to him from this earliest dream.

The Transference.—As the analysis proceeds a change will be noticed in the demeanour of the patient. The ideas that come to the surface, will be projected upon the physician: for instance, should the basis of the neurosis consist in a woman's fixation upon her father, the physician will replace the father in the patient's dream and the repressed erotic impulses will be directed towards the physician, and, since he is not her father the erotic impulses will probably be much less repressed and hidden : or again, if we are dealing with a homosexual patient in like manner the physician becomes the homosexual aim and other ideas and emotions are projected on to him. This transference of the repressed infantile material may take place all at once and may be in the form of great love or its opposite, hate : or it may take place as a series of smaller transferences which reveal individual characteristics. In any case the transference and the dreams connected with it must be analysed in exactly the same manner as the other material, the physician taking care the while to remain quite impersonal, whatever the attitude of the patient to him during this period, which will generally be found to be quite short. When, however, it is explained to him, the patient realises that the impulses and emotions directed towards the father or any other object of his repressed infantile affections have merely been projected upon the physician as substitute, and during the analysis which brings this to the surface the energy behind it all is gradually re-transferred to legitimate objects—in other words—a sublimation is effected. The unconscious conflicts become conscious once the patient faces facts instead of harbouring distorted fancies, and he is cured of his neurotic symptoms.

The physician should throughout the analysis abstain from making up the patient's mind or from giving much advice, and while his attitude should always be thoroughly understanding and sympathetic he should refrain from personal intimacy, and more especially from anything in the nature of physical contact. Personally I never even shake hands with my patients until they are cured and are leaving me. Moreover, should the physician desire to give examples or illustrations on any point it is better for him not to select these from his own life or experience, as the patient's attention is then likely to be taken up by a study of the physician, which wastes time and does not help on the analysis of himself.

One of the essential factors in psycho-analysis is the overcoming of the resistances which prevent the unpleasant material in the subject's mind from becoming conscious. It is often a very disagreeable and very painful process to the patient, and quite as much benefit appears to accrue to the patient as he gradually overcomes this resistance as accrues from the transference or any other part of the analysis. This is why it is of little use to tell the patient what has been discovered until the patient has himself produced such evidence that he can actually realise it consciously. As has already been stated the experienced analyst can often see in a very short time some of the major complexes at the root of a patient's trouble, but it would not be of the slightest use, for instance, to inform a patient that he had an Oedipus complex or an anal-erotic complex, or a homosexual complex. He might very well indeed believe one and accept it as a fact, but accepting that as a scientific fact would have caused him no pain, would have removed nothing from him : it would merely be a diagnosis of his case. The patient must be made to discover these facts for himself, and to overcome the various resistances which prevented them from becoming conscious. I will give an example of what I mean on rather different lines. I have recently had a patient who had completely forgotten the whole of his previous life. He had been invalided from France with shell-shock, and when his parents and his wife visited him he had no recollection of ever having seen them before, but accepted various statements about them and about himself, and finally came to live a fairly normal life, having been told a good deal of his past history. He accepted this also, and indeed knew it to be true, but, as he informed me at his first visit, although he knew it to be true he did not realise the truth by any inner consciousness—*although he knew of past events he did not actually remember them.* After I had hypnotised this man several times and during hypnosis had put him through different epochs in his past life he described a totally different feeling. He now remembered his parents and realised the bond between himself and them, where previously he had merely known them to be his parents : he now remembered facts which he had previously been told and believed in. There was a *realisation* in his mind quite different from the previous *knowledge* and it is a similar realisation which must be sought for in psycho-analysis.

Hence perhaps the reason why psycho-analysis conducted during hypnosis is not always an efficient method of working, because the resistance is done away with in hypnosis and the patient often recalls unpleasant material without any feelings of emotion and then often after a period varying from days to months the resistance may again return. This is not always the case as a patient may without emotion recall under hypnosis early incidents in his life, and after hypnosis one may force them upon the patient's attention, when he may view them with emotion and have to overcome further resistance when discussing them. But this method, so far as I can see, has no advantage over the ordinary method : moreover there are disadvantages in this technique which I know to be carried out by some analysts. The disadvantages are that a considerable proportion of people are not hypnotisable, at any rate not to the point of yielding repressed material verbally during hypnosis, and, that having hypnotised a person one sometimes finds it then much more difficult to analyse him under ordinary conditions. It seems probable that under hypnosis one establishes a form of transference, and possibly to obtain a transference of this kind before one begins analysis forms the barrier to further analysis. At any rate, it is the experience of many analysts, including myself, that when they have hypnotised patients several times the analysis often becomes more difficult, and although on occasion, where a patient is suffering from insomnia or violent headache I may use a little hypnosis, I make it a general rule not to use hypnotism when I am about to analyse. Indeed, I may state that personally I only use hypnotism for three things : insomnia, pain and general amnesia.

As regards the time one should devote to an analysis : the patient should be seen at least four times a week, preferably more often if possible, and as far as possible on consecutive days, because in each gap which is left between the sittings the patient goes through experiences which modify his state of mind, and the smoothness and logical sequence of the analysis is interfered with. About an hour should be devoted to each sitting, though no rule can be made about this. If the patient is in a mood where resistance is at a minimum the analysis should not be broken off because time is up : the next day you may get nothing out of him. On the other hand, if one finds that nothing is being obtained from him and that he is impatient under the analysis, it may be better to discontinue that particular sitting though this is by no means always the case. Resistance seems to vary considerably from day to day, even in discussing the same topic, and resistance manifests itself in many ways.

The unconscious mind of the patient is clever at evading its pursuer, and needs careful watching. For instance, the patient may state that he cannot dream : or he may have so many dreams and such lengthy ones that the whole of the sitting is taken up in discussing their superficial content.

In either case the analyst must not be disturbed. He must not tell the patient to go home until he does remember his dreams, but must select other points which seem suitable and start afresh, or he may tell him to invent a dream, which often does just as well. When the patient finds that he does not avoid analysis by not bringing his dreams he will probably begin to produce them. If the patient dreams too much he should not be allowed to recite all his dreams, but should be stopped when he has reached a certain point and be made to go on with his associations. Another method of evasion is for the patient to give so many associations and so freely, though all of a superficial nature that nothing definite comes out : here the physician must keep bringing the patient back to the point. Again, the patient may state that he has no associations to give : here the physician will point out that the patient cannot have an empty mind, that some ideas must come, and that the patient must catch them as they pass and tell them at once. The whole of the time the physician should be on the alert, watching the patient's expression and movements, and directing the patient's attention to any associations which seem to call forth emotion : but he should never show undue exhilaration when a successful point is made nor disappointment when a long session fails to elicit anything. For it must be borne in mind that very much useless matter is brought to the surface and made much of by the patient's unconscious mind in its attempt to disguise what has been so long repressed.

The associations given by patients vary very much in type. Some will have visual pictures when they close their eyes, and each picture should in turn be analysed in detail, the details usually being reminiscences which may be recent and conscious, or far off in childhood and perhaps forgotten altogether until that moment. Others again have reminiscences without pictures and others may give ideas which come into their heads which are not reminiscences at all but which may be criticisms or judgments arrived at in connection with reminiscences of incidents. Some cases depart altogether from these lines, and when their attention is directed to a dream will simply carry on the dream interminably as a phantasy. I had one patient who would start from his dream and go on for an hour in an apparently aimless fashion in a sort of continuation of the dream : but the material he furnished by this wandering phantasy was so easily translated by the continued repetition of the same situation in a new guise that I rarely disturbed him in his chosen method of association, and indeed his analysis proved to be one of the shortest I have ever undertaken.

As to the time occupied by the analysis it is impossible for the physician to give an definite opinion on this. As a rule a young person of nineteen or twenty has obviously much less material to be unearthed than one who is older and there is less resistance with the former as a rule, though it by no means follows: and I have known cases in which young people could with difficulty be made to speak of themselves at all or even to carry on a conversation. Again, cases of long standing generally take a good deal longer than cases of recent origin, but here it does not follow that there will not be exceptions. I have known a case of sixteen years' standing clear up entirely in two months. Generally speaking, several months must be allowed for an analysis, and cases have been continued by some analysts for a year or two, but I have never had that experience myself. On an average three to six months is long enough to clear up a recent hysteria or compulsion neurosis, though less than three months is by no means uncommon in suitable patients. As regards the suitability of patients it is inadvisable, except in rare instances, to analyse persons over the age of forty-five or fifty years, for such persons have usually become very fixed. In persons of scientific training with plastic minds, however, it is not impossible. The younger the patient, however, the better will be the chance of a successful analysis and quite small children can very easily be analysed. Intelligence and education both render the analysis very much easier, but one can analyse an intelligent person fairly rapidly even though his education be poor : the less intelligence the patient possesses the more difficult will be the analysis. Moreover, if the psychoneurosis is complicated by the presence of any severe organic symptoms the analysis may at times be also more difficult.

Finally, it is recommended that for obvious reasons physicians should not analyse their own relatives. Nor, for a less obvious reason, should they undertake any analysis without taking fees. If a patient be analysed without paying any fee he will take very much longer to analyse because, knowing that if he fails to overcome a resistance on any particular day he can easily put it off till the next day without any further cost, his unconscious mind, ever on the look-out for an excuse to keep up the disguise of his inner feelings, will have a tendency to strengthen the resistance—much as the patient with his conscious mind may desire to be cured : whereas

the mere fact that each successive visit which
is shown to be useless is going to entail an added
cost in the treatment acts as a stimulus to the
breaking down of the resistance.

CHAPTER XII

EXTRACTS FROM THE ANALYSIS OF A COMPULSION NEUROSIS WITH PARANOID SYMPTOMS

THIS case is one of the most suitable for demonstration purposes that I have ever seen, for the following reasons :

1. It was a severe case with marked and definite symptoms, some of which, it is true, bordered upon symptoms of paranoia, but the majority of which comprised an excellent example of the compulsion hysteria.

2. The analysis was extremely straightforward and short, and progressed without a hitch until a complete cure was effected in the short space of about two months.

3. The analysis demonstrated very clearly the mechanism of the formation of a psychoneurosis.

4. The analysis showed well the phenomena of (a) the transference, and (b) the resistances of a typical nature.

With these preliminary remarks I will now pass on to the case itself.

I was called in to see the patient, Miss X., early in October, 19—. Her own doctor was unfortunately unable to be present in consultation, but provided me with a written history of the case of which the following are the essentials. The patient, Miss X., was a woman of thirty-two, of considerable intellectual attainment. On September the 20th (three weeks before I saw her) she had started to do " automatic writing " under some unexplained " compulsion." Four days later she began to hear " voices " speaking to her, details of which were difficult to obtain, but which, though at first merely discursive, gradually assumed a certain amount of persecution.

At the same time the patient became unable to sleep for several nights, and three days later she vomited during the night. The voices continued, and daily became more insistent. The patient became very preoccupied, and was apparently greatly troubled. She complained of severe headache and wept frequently.

On September the 29th she slept during the first part of the night, but woke up in the middle of the night. On the morning of the 30th she was found unconscious in her bed. Upon this Dr. S. was called in and attempted to elucidate the cause of the unconscious condition. Shouting, hard slapping, pricking on the cheek and

soles of the feet and on the hands had no effect
whatever. I am given to understand that
the reaction of the pupils was negligable and
that the corneal reaction was so doubtful that
it could not be claimed. The patient was quite
limp and flaccid, and fell back heavily when
lifted. Dr. S., suspecting hysteria, suggested
an immediate grave operation, but the patient
remained unmoved. Early in the afternoon
consciousness returned, and the doctor stated
that he was unable to say definitely the nature
of the complaint. The patient now spoke quite
normally, and later volunteered information,
about the " automatic writing " and the
" voices." She ate well but looked very ill and
strained. That night again she had no sleep.

The next morning (September 30th) she
looked extremely ill and complained of great
exhaustion, but went to College and lectured
on her customary subjects.

On October 1st she was very exhausted and
preoccupied and answered questions only after
three or four appeals had been made to her.
She was brought home from College in this
condition and put to bed, seemingly very ill
indeed. She became restless, got out of bed,
and wandered about the house. Another doctor, Dr. P., was called in, from whom I had no
report. That night she had no sleep, but

gazed vacantly into space and was very restless.

On October 2nd she was again utterly exhausted. She did not speak and vomited a little. Once or twice she got out of bed and wandered. She was quiet and amenable, but had an abnormal facial expression. Her eyes are described as " glaring," and she kept throwing her head back and smiling. She also began to bite at her sheets. Occasionally, in answer to questions, she answered " yes " or " no " at random, although she knew everybody and reacted almost normally to visitors for a short time, apparently with very great effort. Dr. S. visited her again but was doubtful as to what course to take with her. She was quiet and may have had some sleep during this night.

On October 3rd she appeared a little better and managed to sleep.

On October 4th the improvement continued somewhat ; she still, however, insisted on doing automatic writing, and complained that the voices were almost continuous, and that they were of a persecutory nature. The question of her sanity was discussed, but fortunately for the patient no decision was arrived at then and there.

On the next day I myself visited the patient who was still in bed, and was able to hold a long and satisfactory conversation with her, but before going into this part of the case I must add a few further words on her own medical history in order to complete the picture.

The patient's general health was fairly good, although she occasionally suffered from neuralgia. Her menstrual periods were regular, but she suffered great pain, which often caused nausea and vomiting. The actual flow was excessive, and extended frequently over one week. Eight years previously she had had an operation in hospital, which she described as " being scraped out "—probably a curetting. This improved her condition somewhat. In August, 19—, *a few days before her mental trouble began, she saw a well-known gynæcologist, who examined her* but found nothing organically wrong, and suggested that the pain might be due to habit.

With regard to the family history, both her father and her younger brother were normal, but her mother was at one time ill for eight years with " internal tumours." No operation was performed, and in time the tumour disappeared. Simultaneously with the disappearance of the tumour her mind became affected. She was in an asylum for about three years, then was well for two years, but a relapse occurred in July, 19—, when she seemed at times insane (*this was about one month before my patient developed her neurosis)*; she was not, however, again sent to an asylum. At this time the father was fifty-six years old, the mother sixty years old, and the brother twenty-five.

I will now pass on to my first visit to the patient. She was in bed and appeared to be very weak and exhausted, but her expectations with regard to me having been raised somewhat high, she was very pleased to see me and anxious to tell about her condition.

I made a fairly comprehensive examination of her reflexes and sensations and found nothing abnormal. On this occasion I led her to talk about her alleged " trance," and she admitted that she was conscious during the whole period of her examination, but that something within her told her that she must not wake up but must lie still and passive whatever were done. This was apparently confirmed by voices which spoke to her, but her memory on this latter point was not very good. The only other points which I gleaned from her at this visit were that she was almost continuously worried by voices, some of which she recognised as friends—one killed in the war—others of strangers. These latter were often of a persecutory nature. Further, she was quite certain that the voices were real and were not hallucinations. She also told me that she was convinced that the automatic writing had come from " the other side." Lastly, I gathered that a group of living people, namely, *thirty-two* members of the Psychical Society, were at enmity with her. She also stated that she had recently read " Raymond " by Sir Oliver Lodge.

I did not attempt to persuade her that she was the victim of hallucinations, but assured her that I understood the condition quite well ; that there was no need for her to stay in bed ; and that for purposes of treatment she would have to visit me in future. I then persuaded her to get up and have tea in her dining room and then left her.   I mention all these facts merely to show that one does not suddenly plunge into any sudden form of psycho-analysis, but that sympathy and tact may form a very essential preliminary stage : sometimes this must be continued over a somewhat prolonged period.

During her next two visits to me I did not attempt any analysis, but contented myself with explaining the nature of psycho-analysis and with gradually eliciting something of her family life and sexual history.

Her sexual history elicited at this stage was as follows : at the age of three she had accidentally (so far as she remembered) discovered the pleasure of masturbation, and had practised this fairly regularly ever since. She did not know whether there was an interval after the age of three when she had temporarily left off the practice.

I very frequently "break in" the patient to analysis by means of the word association test, but in this case I had such a wealth of material to go on and the patient was anxious to plunge into the midst of her troubles, so I started upon analysis of the automatic writing. Before doing this I impressed upon her the fact that though the writing, the voices and other items of persecution might seem quite real to her, yet for the purpose of analysis she must for the time being imagine them to be products of her unconscious mind, and treat them as such." Space will not permit me to go into the complete analysis of the automatic writing, especially as I wish to quote the apparently purposeless portions as well as those of analytical value, in order to demonstrate how much trivial matter one must patiently contend with in order to obtain any useful material. I will therefore quote a portion only of the writing, which led to certain facts being forthcoming. It started as follows : (The writing purported to have come from a spirit and was interspersed with Miss X.'s comments and questions, also in writing; the two handwritings were quite different) :

The Spirit. (Illegible words). " . . . . to write. Have you read the sentence, my darling ? "

Miss X. " No, not the first part."

The Spirit. " Why do you want to write ? "

Miss X. " I want to know things about spiritual life in other spheres than this. I am seriously interested in them, but I do not want to do anything wicked or wrong."

The Spirit. " You only want to know for curiosity."

Miss X. " I suppose it is chiefly that: also I want to be convinced of the existence of spirits. I think I am, and I believe it is a serious and real thing to be convinced of, but I am not quite sure. I should like to know if people go on living after they are dead."

The Spirit. " What are . . . . " (Rest illegible).

Miss X. " Will you write that again ? "

The Spirit. " What are Magdalene's moods ? "

Miss X.	" Who are you and what do you mean ? "
The Spirit.	" Darling, I am your lover. I died years ago, my darling, my angel."
Miss X.	" How can you be ? Did you ever know me ? "
The Spirit.	" Why not ? "
Miss X.	" I have never had a lover that I know of."
The Spirit.	" Yes."
Miss X.	" What is your name ? "
The Spirit.	" My name is William Morris, my own."
Miss X.	" When did you know me ? "
The Spirit.	" Mine own wife you are. I met you in Sunny Spain, my darling. I love you."
Miss X.	" Was I your wife in the life I lived previous to this ? "
The Spirit.	" Yes, you were, my darling."
Miss X.	" Shall I be anyone else's wife in this life, or do I still belong to you ? "
The Spirit.	" You are going to marry another man soon."
Miss X.	" How soon ? "
The Spirit.	(Answer illegible.)
Miss X.	" Can't you tell me ? "

The Spirit. " Nine months: you are going
to be engaged in a fortnight.
You will meet him to-morrow
in the Tube."

Miss X. " Thank you for telling me. Will
you tell me some more about
how I shall meet him, so that I
may know that what you say is
true ? "

The Spirit. " You *must* believe."

Miss X. " If what you say comes true,
then I am bound to believe."

The Spirit. " You do believe."

Miss X. " Yes, I think so."

The Spirit. " I, . . . (words illegible), my
darling, my own."

Miss X. " Are you sorry I am going to be
married to another man ? "

The Spirit. " Yes."

Miss X. " Are you in this life now, as I
am ? Or are you a spirit ? "

The Spirit. " I am a spirit."

Miss X. " Where are you living ? "

The Spirit. " In Heaven."

Miss X. " Are you happy ? "

The Spirit. " Yes."

Miss X. " Do you like talking to me like
this ? "

The Spirit. " Yes."

Miss X.	" Is it right to do it ? "
The Spirit.	" Yes."
Miss X.	" Is it dangerous ? "
The Spirit.	" Yes."
Miss X.	" For me or for you ? "
The Spirit.	" For you, because you may get hurt by evil spirits which may come into communication with you."
Miss X.	" How can I guard against the evil ones ? "
The Spirit.	" You must pray as you do it."
Miss X.	" Is it all right now ? "
The Spirit.	" Yes."
Miss X.	" Why ? "
The Spirit.	" Because you prayed."
Miss X.	" You mean before I began to-night ? "
The Spirit.	" Yes."
Miss X.	" If you are in Heaven and are happy, why do you mind if I marry again ? "
The Spirit.	" Because you are going to be another's. You will meet him at the Tube, on the station, at Baker Street. He will meet you at the Booking Office. You will meet him in the queue. He will say : ' Can you soon marry me? ' "

Miss X.   " Shall I be too shocked to answer ? "

The Spirit. " No ! "

Miss X.   " Is he a good and nice man ? "

The Spirit. " Yes."

Miss X.   " Is he a soldier ? "

The Spirit. " Yes."

Miss X.   " What shall I say to him ? "

The Spirit. " You will say, ' Wait a little . . . (words illegible).' "

Miss X.   " What comes after ' Wait a little ' ? "

The Spirit. " Why act so soon ? "

Miss X.   " Do I know the man already ? "

The Spirit. " No."

Miss X.   " Then it will be love at first sight for both of us ? "

The Spirit. " Yes."

Miss X.   " What is his name ? "

The Spirit. " William Moore."

There were many dozens of pages following this, which continued daily and purported to be descriptions of the condition of spirits on the other side. There were also messages purporting to come from Raymond Lodge and a man called Charles Yasting. But the essential part of my analysis of the automatic writing was concerned with the portion I have quoted.

It would be interesting, but unnecessary, to

go into the whole of it. I may add that Miss X., on being informed by the spirit of the hour at which she was to go to the station to meet her unknown lover, actually *did* go there, but he failed to keep the appointment. She came back and accused the spirit of having misled her, but he pointed out that it was entirely her fault as she was a few minutes late at the trysting place.

The spirit's handwriting throughout was quite different from that of Miss X., and there is no doubt that while writing she was quite unconscious of what the alleged spirit was going to say and was quite convinced that she was in communication with someone who had previously died. I now pass on to the analysis of a few portions of this writing.

I said: " Give me some associations to: " *The name, William Morris.*"

She replied: " A poet—is connected with automatic writing—also with William Moore. This brings to mind the fact that I stopped the writing at one stage because William Morris said I was to. Billy. Charles Yasting. His wife. College. Botany. Cultures. Research work. . . . ." (A long pause.)

" *Yes ; go on.*"

" Nothing. I can't."

" *Go on,*" I urged.

" Googlywogs.   Rot.   Fathead.   Silly.   This is rot."

(This sample shows how unpromising an analysis may seem, especially to the beginner).

Then followed a good deal of similar matter, most of which was unimportant. I took her back to the word " Googlywogs," and asked her to explain that.

Googlywogs.—" Careless—happy and flippant."

Goo.—" Bergoo, a name for porridge we had in childhood.   We didn't like it.   Food : war rations."

Googly.—" O Lord !   What have I done to you ? Sugar.   Something sweet—through bergoo —and sugar on porridge.   I used to give mine to the dog.   (Pause.)   I don't know any more."

Wogs.—" A dog—a little one we have—Jacky— another name for him is Wiggle-Waggle. Love—she's rather a nice dog.   It makes me feel as if someone were telling me they were in love with me."   (Pause.)

" *Yes.   How do you connect that with dog ?* "
  ' " Shouldn't think there is much connection. Perhaps their sexual intercourse.   I used to be interested in it as a child. . .   Sugar sticks : we used to have rabbits in the garden.   The dogs teased them.   Rabbits : I've looked out of the window at them while

I've been ill. I've connected them in my mind with myself. I don't know how: they remind me of the calf in the book of Revelations."

"*The calf ?*"

"It's symbolic : a sacrifice. I had to sacrifice myself, although I was doing something very silly, to help on something I know nothing about."

"*Yes ?*"

"Psychical Research. I had to sacrifice myself to defend people from something very wrong. I won't tell you what."

"*Yes. Go on.*"

"No, I won't."

"*William Morris : get back to him again.*"

"He was a poet : he wrote a poem—I forget it's name : begins with a P. The lines at the end of it. . . I forget them. O yes, the poem is called 'Prospice.'" (Here is an excellent example of resistance causing forgetting).

"*That poem is by Browning,*" I replied, "*and the last lines are these :*

"Then a light
Then thy breast, O thou soul of my soul,
I shall clasp thee again
And with God be the rest !*"

At this point Miss X. blushed deeply and

showed considerable emotion, indicating, as indeed does the whole automatic writing, a repressed desire to " clasp " somebody—*i.e.*, a repressed erotic desire towards the male sex.

A few more similar analytic points led to the same conclusion, and I asked Miss X. if she did not agree with this. I pointed out that she was of a marriageable age, exceptionally good-looking, intelligent, and asked if there were any reason why she should repress this desire for marriage. She said that she thought that on several occasions the opportunity might have arisen, but that curiously enough she could not bear a man to touch her in any way. As soon as it reached the point that a man might put his arm round her waist she was filled with an immediate horror and everything was " off " at once. She could assign no reason for this state of affairs, so I left the matter for the time being and took up my thread with the next name that occurred in the automatic writing.

" *Magdalene's Moods ?* "

" Magdalene. A woman : Christ forgave her her sins. Cutting up bluebell stalks. Pretending to be the Virgin Mary—just happy and placid—submissive—silly—cutting off dead ends of flowers. I was doing this when I had to say I was she—the

Virgin Mary—The Dream of Gerontius—a poem."

"*The Virgin Mary—go back to that.*"

"I felt I was the Virgin Mary before I had the trance—I believed I was the Virgin Mary. In the trance I thought there was a spirit in the room. The Virgin Mary conceived of the Holy Ghost." (Here Miss X. looked confused and angry, and it was with greater difficulty that I persuaded her to proceed.)

"*The Virgin Mary.*"

"The Holy Spirit—anger—feeling angry— I was the Holy Spirit as well as the Virgin Mary—but at different times. I had to be angry and find out things that were wrong." (Pause.)

"*Yes?*"

"Things that were wrong with work— things that were wrong with the Psychical Research Society."

"*Yes.*"

"The Virgin Mary is not like me." It will be observed that Miss X. very promptly left the "Psychical Research Society" owing to resistance and returned to a less resistant point, though it was one that led to a good deal of information being given.

"I am wicked. The Virgin Mary was pure." Here was her obvious "wish" expression in assuming the part of the Virgin Mary in her hysteria. Moreover, the Virgin Mary was enabled to conceive without having to touch any man—a thing Miss X. detested. Here again is the " wish " expressed in excellent symbolism.

I asked Miss X. if she accepted this explanation and she replied that it had already occurred to her a few minutes previously. It was further borne out at a later stage of the proceedings.

I am now going to leave out a good deal of the analysis of the automatic writing—much of it was wandering and apparently far from the point ; I say " apparently," for no doubt the irrelevant matter really constituted a long chain of associations. I wish to give such portions of the analysis as clearly demonstrate the facts of this case, and at the same time to give a fair proportion of so-called irrelevant matter ; but many of the facts which came to light did so on various occasions and through different channels of association, and it is not my intention to give all these redundant facts.

The next part of the analysis of paramount interest was that connected with the " Psychical Research Society."

I must here explain that Miss X. shared a flat with another woman friend of about her own age. This lady, whom I will call Miss Yates, gave me the following precis of a statement made by Miss X. during the height of her illness, Miss X. being highly excited and insistent throughout.

"The Psychical Research Society is doing something terribly wrong. It is injuring people—doing horrid things to them. (Miss Yates asked: 'To people you know?') Yes (mentioning names) and to others who have lost people in the war. (Miss Yates asked what injuries). The injuries are of a sexual nature. (Details were not given to me by Miss Yates). They will come and tell me so. Will they come to-night? There are *thirty-two** of them. They must come to-night. They must come before I can go to sleep. They injure others as they injured me when you were away. They did things to me in the night and made me ill. I help the people they injure by praying. I have helped some : these will come and tell me so. They used me as F—— (the medium in 'Raymond') my subconscious self. You were there too. I must help by praying and in some other way—I don't know what. I have to fight against evil : it makes me ill, but it may be worth while. They use me to injure others—I have to fight against it by praying. They tried

<hr>

Associations to "32" at once gave "My age—32 years of wasted life—bad life.' The members of the S.P.R. apparently represented her own *conscious* research into her psychic life of the previous 32 years—which had been taking place just previous to her illness.

to injure you : I said I wouldn't have you in. They will come and tell you."

Miss X. was thoroughly convinced of the reality of this persecution : there was no doubt of that.

Now as the analysis of the Psychical Research Society I will only give, as before, portions that are relevant to an understanding of the case.   I asked for associations :

" *The Psychical Research Society ? "*

> " Raymond—spirits—once when I went away for a holiday I played a game with a tumbler that spelled out words, and someone did automatic writing."

(Here followed matter which did not at the moment lead anywhere, and I left it for the time being.)

" *The Psychical Research Society again ? "*

> " They are terribly wrong, injuring people by letting husbands and wives communicate after the husband is dead. The medium might take part of a personality and use it through the spirit. Also they do sexual injuries."

" *Yes.—They injured you. ?*

> " I felt things in the dark. . . ."

" *Yes ? "*

> " I don't know what I mean."

" *Go on."*

(Miss X., however, stopped here and went on to another point, so I reserved this one for future use. It is no use wasting time on a thread the patient will not follow. It is better to return to it when other information has come out elsewhere.) Miss X. continued:

" After I went to meet the man at the Tube I went on writing, and voices directed me to do things. I was still in bed. The people I helped by prayer were shocked. The voices told me so. I spoke to the Psychical Research Society about it and then I came to a full stop because they did not listen. Voices made me go and meet the man again on Sunday. He wasn't there. In the night when I was in a trance I had an uncomfortable experience, as if someone were in the room in the dark. I had sensations as if one were married. I imagined it was a spirit. I think it was Christ, I am not sure. Then afterwards I thought it was my dead friend, Yastings. I heard them speaking; they talked about religion as though they were making love. They wanted me to stay in bed and told me I must not wake up. I imagined the spirit was in bed with me, but it turned into a man. Then I got a sensation."

" Do you mean a normal sexual sensation?" I asked

" I do not know if I was quite satisfied
sexually. Next day they fetched the doctor
and I wouldn't wake up. I have had normal
sexual sensations often when awake, but
not before in a trance. In a dream I have.
Years back I had such feelings in my dreams.
I was 25 or 26 ; but these feelings were not
complete."

This portion of the analysis again shows
very clearly that Miss X. had strong sexual
desires which were repressed ; that the idea of
sexual relationship with a man was desired and
repressed ; and it bears out our previous finding
that she could not bear a man to touch her. It
is obvious then that she was not of a true homosexual nature in her unconscious—though
superficially she would appear to be so, and even
physically she appeared superficially to be so,
as we shall find shortly.

Free association was continued from the last
point, viz. : the sexual dreams of the patient,
which were incomplete. She continued :

" I have had complete satisfaction when
awake very frequently, but not lately.
Lately I have tried not to do it. The first
time must have been at about the age of
three or four years. I found it out for
myself. I have done things with other
girls ; I can still see them—the girls. I

have never had anything to do with a man
sexually " (Pause.)

" Yes ? " I urged her.

" The last time I masturbated was when
I was ill in bed ; about the time I had my
trance, but before that I must have been
three or four months without anything of
the kind."

Later on, out of another series of analyses which
I need not go into fully, a continuation of the
sexual history took place, as follows :

" I have only masturbated at rare intervals
during the last two years ; but previously
I used to do it once or twice a week. About
three months ago I did it with another
girl."

" Why did you fight against your desires recently? "

" It was not good for me. I have felt very
passionate, but have resisted it. I think
one oughtn't to do it. It is wrong. After
doing it I have felt guilty. It is distasteful
to me. I have been more religious lately
since my trance ; before that my religion
(Church of England), was of a very unemo-
tional type. Now it is different since all
this happened."

Here we have a good example of a sublimation
of psychic energy, from a sexual emotion to a
religious emotion. This has been brought about

by the patient herself in an attempt to defend herself from the unbearable ideas.

I used to have a report from the friend, Miss Yates, with whom Miss X. shared her flat. I will quote a few notes from this about this period in order to demonstrate that up to the present very little had really been accomplished; we had only begun to gather our different threads together.

Fragments of daily report :

> *October 18th and 19th.*—Very abstracted. Did a few household tasks, some wrong, very slowly: Laughed frequently.
>
> *October 20th.*—Same as above. Played piano a little, fairly well. On being questioned talked to me quite freely about the voices, and insisted that she *knew* that she was talking with other people's subconscious selves about religion and such things, and it was very important that she should do so. She had found out how to do it and was learning how to help. It was more important than anything else. She told me some facts the voices had told her about one of my friends, which I was able to prove quite incorrect.
>
> *October 21st.*—Very restless and tired ; seemed more abstracted. Reads a little (very little actual reading, I think) ; Thompson's

" Poems," " Atonement and Personality,"
by Moberly, " The Treasure of the Hum-
ble," by Maeterlinck, and the " Differential
Calculus." She lies awake a long time after
going to bed and wakes early in the morning.
Remembers very little of what happens,
although her mind is quite clear about events
before she started the automatic writing.

October 23rd.—Complains of feeling giddy
when she walks and when she tries to attend
much to outside things or conversation.
Says she now understands non-Euclidean
Geometry.

It will be clear from this that the voices which
spoke to her were still in the nature of delusions ;
that they had not yet become hallucinations, a
stage commonly found as this type of hysteria
clears up.

Out of these daily reports I used occasionally
to obtain material for association, and from this
set in particular I laid bare one repressed mental
conflict. I asked for some association to the
" Differential Calculus, to which Miss X. seemed
very partial at this time, and obtained the
following :

" *Differential Calculus :* Mathematics ;
education ; my ambitions ; I desire to
become a great educationalist—not merely
a teacher—a principal and a pioneer in

education. I have not thought about this
lately ; it used to be a very great ambition."

" *Yes ? Why have you not thought about it
lately ?* "

" I don't know."

" *Did you ever have other ambitions ?* "

" Yes. I longed above all things to have a
house of my own and a husband and children. I want real family life."

" *Well ?* "

" It is not possible to have that and also
to become a great educationalist—besides,
I don't think I shall ever marry."

" *I see,*" said I. " *The two ideals, the educational
one on the one hand and the family ideal on the
other, are in your mind incompatible ?* "

" Yes."

" *So,*" I continued, " *you repressed the conflict
between the two, which was insoluble, and added
its force to other repressions causing your
Neurosis.*"

She seemed quite pleased with this solution,
and stated that she felt sure that it was true. I
pointed out that she must definitely take one
path or another in all such cases, instead of
repressing the conflict, even if afterwards she
changed her mind and choose another path. I
introduce this small portion of the analysis as
being an example of the many mental conflicts

which may be repressed and which, though in themselves insufficient to cause a hysteria, may add the sum of their force to others and have effect in its final determination.

A return to the analysis of the automatic writing about this period led to some important details being given which were not entirely forgotten, but which had hitherto been hidden from me, partly out of loyalty to the patient's friend, Miss Yates. I will just quote one of the important portions.

" *Associations to the name Charles Yastings ?* "

" His wife ; he's a decent fellow. I stayed with them after they were married. I went to say goodbye to her at the station. She didn't like me smiling at her husband. She thought I meant more than I did. I meant nothing. She was at college with me ; a good friend. I never did anything sexual with her."

" *Why do you add that last sentence ?* "

" I don't know ; it came into my mind."

" *Well, go on with Charles Yastings.* "

" His was one of the first voices I heard. He wrote in the automatic writing and talked to me. When I was digging he talked of things I was doing. He also talked to me in the theatre when the play was going on ; nothing important. He wanted me to write to his wife. He wanted me to stop writing because it was dangerous. I was friendly with them both. He said he was desperate in my life. I don't know what he meant."

" Why should he have come to you ? "

" Because he is the only man I knew well who was dead. I don't know many men well." Then she continued: " Yastings sounds like Yates (the friend's name with whom Miss X. lived). I am more friendly with her. . . I was not in love with Charles Yastings; I've never been in love with a man. I've never had passionate feelings towards a man——. Yes, once, about four months ago: in a railway carriage—a stranger; by accident he was exposing a little of his body and I felt passionate then."

It will be noticed that even this incident did not revive similar childish memories which we shall discover later on.

She went on: " I've never been proposed to; I've never really been in love: my two greatest loves have been my mother and Miss Yates."

" Which is the greater love ? "

" Miss Yates; I've been in love with another girl, too, before."

" Yes—go on."

" Now I have no affection for Miss Yates.
When she went to stay away I was alone.
She doesn't like seeing people or going out.
I do ; but I had to go with her only. I
think you may call it ' being in love.' I
used to have sexual pleasures with her, but
I couldn't get any pleasure unless I imagined
she was a man."

Here we see again that in spite of homosexual
actions, psychically Miss X. is not a homosexual,
nor is she in any way " inverted." As yet we
have no evidence, however, as to why she has
this " pseudo-homosexual " complex.

I now pass on to a dream which occurred at a
somewhat later date. I did not do a full analysis
of the dream for two reasons, firstly because the
one point analysed gave us the essential facts,
and secondly because at the next sitting we had
to enter into other matters that had arisen.
Several other short dreams were analysed, each
giving their small quota to the investigation, but
space will not permit me to give all the details,
nor is it necessary to the understanding of the
case.

The Dream.

" Some one—a woman, I think—took a
photograph out of an envelope which was
lying on my desk and gave the photograph
to me to look at. It was a group of girls

whom I did not know, and I thought the
name of one of them was a Welsh name.
Then I woke up."

I asked for associations to the Welsh name.

" The name that comes into my head," said
Miss X., " is Jenny Phillips, a girl I was at
school with. We used to travel to school
in the train together.":

" *How old were you ?* "

" Eight or nine years old." (Pause.)

" *Go on.*"

The patient was considerably agitated and
looked very pained. She stated that she
could not remember any more, but on being
further urged, continued : " Several of us
used to travel to school in the train together.
There was often a man in the train. I'd
forgotten all about him until now, or I'd
have told you before. He used to read a
newspaper, and beneath the newspaper he
used to open his trousers and expose his
genital organs to us. One day when I was
alone, and getting out of the carriage, he
put his hand up my skirt as I passed. I
was terribly frightened and told the school
mistress. There was a fearful row about
it all. It's funny, but I've quite forgotten
the whole thing until this minute."

" *Does it throw any light on your condition ?* "

" Yes.   I'm quite sure that my fear of men touching me dates from that time, now I think of it."

After a little thought she then explained to me that she could now see how this fact had given her a horror of contact with men, although she wished to be married, and that no doubt this was why she had behaved in a homosexual fashion and had yet been obliged to imagine that the other woman was a man.

I did not have to explain or point out any of these facts to her.

On the next visit I was pleased to find a very great improvement.   The voices were fewer and less insistent, and moreover were now recognised as hallucinations.   Miss X. realised at last that she had had delusions, but that the voices now were quite unreal.   However, I was annoyed to find that she had developed another symptom, which we had to do a short analysis of.   She complained that she felt a tight band round her head.   I asked her to concentrate her mind on it and tell me what came into her mind.,

" Trying to read Pfister—that was the first time—the snakes—windows—trying to see the connection between different interpretations .in Pfister.   Bands—the speckled band of Holmes—bell ropes—trying to remember things—the iron clamp of a retort stand—working in a laboratory. I get it when I try to recall scenes from my early life. It tightens up then. I feel as if I were looking in my head for something. I I think of elastic bands and father's shop and father. Something whirling round— the band is like that—a flat disc with a big hole in the centre—like a halo whirling round—a tight halo—Neptune—I don't see what it symbolises unless I take for granted Pfister's interpretation of snakes and male symbols, and that doesn't seem the right interpretation. It's like a halo."

" *What does a halo symbolise ? "*

" A saint—good people—angels."

" *Yes. And have you not recently represented one?"*

" You mean the Virgin Mary ? Of course ; well, what does it mean then ? Oh ! it's the same thing, of course."

I pointed out to her what I wish now to point out to my readers that very often when one hysterical sign disappears under treatment another replaces it if the analysis has not completely removed the repressed complexes. Obviously here the remnants of her repression were still at work, and brought out this new symptom —to wit, wearing a halo instead of being the Virgin Mary. The symptom disappeared that day and did not recur.

We had now cleared up the major causes of the neurosis, at any rate the symptoms had suddenly cleared up, and the causation of them was recognised by the patient as lying in the repressed material which had come to light. The dreams which were now reported to me indicated clearly that the Transference was the next thing which we must analyse. As I have before pointed out, during an analysis the energy of the repressed desires gets transferred to the physician, and the patient in this condition, though possibly free from hysterical symptoms, is now perhaps very fond of the physician and inclined to rely upon his judgment and help in all things—a state of affairs which must not be allowed to remain as a permanent fixation. In other words the " transference " must be analysed and the repressed energy sublimated, or turned into other and useful channels. The patient brought me the following dream :

"I was in a small room of which I could see one wall only—straight in front of me. A shutter in the wall opened and a man from the outside rolled in a bright tin can. And then the shutter closed up and it was dark again."

I asked her emotions during the dream and she replied that they were of pleased interest.

To my mind this was obviously a dream belonging to the transference, and I asked her to give me a few associations, which were as follows :

" *The room ?* "

> " It symbolises my mind—a large space—darkness and stars—sky at night—the shutter in a shop—a butcher's shop—joints of meat on hooks and a man with a blue apron on. The room was dark—nothing in it—empty—photography—doing experiments —on light—I know what it means : the room represents my mind ; the tin can is a symbol of hypnotism—the mirror you use. *You* were the man outside. It represented the idea of hypnotic suggestion by you, and the suggestion stayed in my mind when the shutter was shut."

I had used hypnotism on two occasions to assist sleep for Miss X., as she had been so troubled with insomnia.

" *The tin can ?* "

> " I rather liked the tin can being inside, because I thought it was something interesting."

" *The open shutter ?* "

> " A panel—something to slide up and down —the door open in Heaven—a camera."

" *The man.*" '

> " Stooping—the shutter wasn't wide

enough—medium size—fairly thin—ordinary clothes—no hat. It was you of course helping me. . . . " (Pause).

"*Put your mind on the man.*"

"He's different now. I see in his hands a rolling pin. He's strange now. I don't think I know him. God is Love—all doors are open to Him."

"*A bright tin can?*"

"A Jersey milk can—one I have on the piano that my brother sent me. Hypnotism. It was a cylindrical can, and I thought it was empty. It was brightly polished—milk—cradles for babies—feeding bottles. The time when I was small and took my brother's feeding bottle from him and sucked at it myself when mother wasn't there."

"*Yes. Go on.   *"

"Rolling* and bicycling. Cycling down hill. Rolling pennies down an inclined plane. The principle of Archimedes. Eureka—loss of weight—me having a bath—it suggests the man in a bath and the bath flowing over."

These associations, as well as the dream, are obviously entirely sexual, but analysis would

*The word rolling is here twice repeated and is a significant association on account of her previous reference to a rolling pin.

get no further than her previous statement, that the room was her brain, I was the man, the shutters of the room opening represented the opening of her mind to receive the good which was represented by the bright can.

Now I knew that the essential translation had not yet come to the surface, owing to the resistance she was offering. I was unwilling to tell her the meaning of the dream and asked her to think it over at home and tell me on the next day if she could make anything else out of it.

Meanwhile I had lunch with a friend and told him of this dream and translated it as follows : The room was her own reproductive organs ; the man was myself ; the bright can was the male reproductive organ. This was confirmed by the fact that she afterwards saw the man with a rolling-pin in his hand, an obvious phallic symbol. In other words the dream represented repressed and unconscious erotic desires towards the analyst.

On the next day she came and informed me that she had found the meaning of the dream. She said : " It is a sex dream in which the room would symbolise the womb, and the tin can would symbolise the male organ, and the shutter the vagina—the brightness of the tin can a desire for purity in the man." I asked her who was the man, and she said *she had not the vaguest idea*. I asked her what man held the rolling-pin and she told me that *she did not remember any rolling-pin and had not mentioned one*. This is an excellent example of the resistance forcing unpleasant truths into the background. I then asked her who was the man she had suggested in the translation she gave me yesterday. " *Oh you !* " she exclaimed, and for a moment seemed quite upset. I soon, however, explained the nature of transference to her and she was at once quite at ease.

I have said very little about the actual stimuli which determined the final onset of the neurosis, but no doubt the following facts had a considerable bearing on the matter. The patient, though very fond of her mother, was always troubled in mind when at home with her, for Miss X. was educated far beyond her mother's standard. A month before the onset of the neurosis the mother had a relapse into her previous state of mental instability, and during Miss X.'s visits at home she had to treat her mother as a child and look after her : at other times the mother was quite sane and treated Miss X. as a child : the consequence was, after every visit home at a week-end, Miss X., who at the time was very much overworked, was reduced to tears and felt very ill. Nor must it be overlooked that her menstrual pains had caused her to go to a gynæcologist a few days before the onset of her trouble, and no doubt his physical examination, questions, and so forth, all touched upon the repressed complexes concerning contact with men and tended to make the repression ineffectual. As a defence against these things becoming conscious Miss X. developed her hysteria.*

A few more sittings completed the case and she was perfectly well and happy. The last I heard of her was that she felt better and happier than she had ever done before and that she was glad she had had her illness, as the analysis had helped her to understand herself and life in general in a way in which she had not before deemed possible.

I have given many trivial details in this case in order to show how many apparently foolish and trivial matters creep in during an analysis; how it often looks as though nothing would ever become clear; but how, by following first one thread and then another we can at length get down to the causation of a trouble.

Moreover this case is very complete and exemplifies several points remarkably well:

(1). The reasons for a particular series of

*Miss X showed a strong father fixation, and a great jealousy at times towards her mother.

symptoms appearing, namely, the idea of conception and sexual pleasure without the intervention of man.

(2) The change of a symptom from one form to another as the analysis clears away some of the repressions, *e.g.*, in the substitution of a halo for the previous idea of the Virgin Mary.

(3) The resistances that we find, and particularly the complete forgetting of recent events and thoughts, *e.g.*, in the analysis of the transference dream resistance caused the patient to forget important details she had given the day before.

(4) The transference itself is well exemplified.

(5) We see clearly the repression of insoluble conflicts and the expression of repressed wishes in the hysteria itself.

To the experienced analyst many other points are apparent throughout this analysis, which space does not permit one to go into fully here. There was a strongly marked Electra complex, there was sexual aggression in infancy well marked in two ways, namely, early masturbation, and acts of cruelty to her young brother, etc., etc. The object of this chapter is not so much to give a full analysis of the case—which would occupy a whole volume—as to illustrate the maze of material through which one must wander, and the methods by which one can finally arrive at the underlying complexes.

CHAPTER XIII

SOME CRITICISMS OF PSYCHO-ANALYSIS

A GREAT many criticisms have been levelled against psycho-analysis, and in all cases, so far as I have been able to see, by people who have never taken the trouble to study the subject thoroughly. They have perhaps read one book on the subject, or on one branch of the subject and then without further thought have made criticisms which any one conversant with psycho-analysis knows at once to be based upon a total misconception of the subject from first to last. Exactly the same took place when Darwin first propounded his theory of evolution, and the reason in both cases is not far to seek. Everyone likes to have a good opinion of himself; he looks upon himself with lenient eyes, and anything that at once shows that his pride in himself is thoroughly unjustified is cast away with anger and scorn. Man rationalises everything; if he be a total abstainer he will bring what seems to him absolute proof that alcohol is the invention of the devil. If he be a drinker

269

of alcohol in small measure, then he will justify that by equally plausible reasoning. If he be a Roman Catholic, he will show quite clearly that this is the only religion which may safely steer any man to Heaven while a member of some other church will, with apparently infallible logic, show that the Pope and all Popish things are wiles of the devil. That which we wish to prove we rationalise and, working from imperfect premises, we prove to ourselves to be true. Hence, when Darwin showed that our bodies were not created suddenly by divine interposition but that they were developed from a lower form of life, the insult to man's blatant belief in himself and his infallible position in the universe was too great. It created that which we have discussed in previous chapters, namely, a strong *resistance*. The proofs of the unpleasant material were at once repressed, and for a short period, having rationalised the matter, man placidly believed his pleasant lies. The same has happened in respect of other novel ideas which once were scorned and which now are accepted, and the same occurs in many people with regard to psycho-analysis. Psychoanalysis shows them that they are not the perfect creatures which they had supposed themselves to be. It shows the saint that he still possesses sex in his unconscious mind, possibly displaced, possibly sublimated; possibly it shows him that he is a sexual pervert. It shows the woman of fashion that in many ways she is but a barbarian with an infantile mind. The resistance, the same internal resistance which is met with during every psychoanalysis, prevents these people from even examining a subject, lest the truth should be unpleasant for them. Everywhere and everywhen they rationalise.

These then are some of the reasons which prevented psycho-analysis from gaining at once the position which it must eventually hold and is steadily achieving. However, there are an increasing number of people, educated and open-minded, who are anxious not only to find the truth at any cost but to see the world progressing and to see the evil in it, however pleasant, sublimated into something which may be just as pleasant yet not so deleterious; so that psycho-analysis has now obtained a firm footing and an ever widening circle of earnest and scientific students. One or two specific objections which I have recently heard may perhaps be mentioned here with advantage.

Several people have said to me: " Psychoanalysis is excellent, but it lacks anything spiritual." They seem to think that in benefiting the mind of a person one must deal with spiritual things. My reply is: " Chemical analysis also lacks anything spiritual, and indeed so does almost every form of analysis." From its very nature analysis consists merely in a scientific and precise investigation into the component parts of any thing or subject. Such questioners do not realise the true meaning of analysis and they are apt to assume that psycho-analysis destroys religion. In this they are absolutely wrong, for the psycho-analyst recognises that all forms of religion are for many patients valuable channels of sublimation and he would no more think of trying to disturb a patient's religion than a physician would of trying to disturb his patient's digestion. Moreover the findings of psycho-analysis do not upset religious ideas any more than Darwin's findings in physical evolution, though like Darwin the psycho-analyst may upset many of the non-essential formulæ and dogmas. Indeed, one of the chief things which psycho-analysis has done has been merely to show that like the body the mind has evolved, but that as in the body many primitive, rudimentary and at present useless factors are present, and that in the psychical as well as in the physical plane of humanity evolution is still proceeding.

The second difficulty which many people find is in the theory of determinism, in which

Freud himself, the originator of psycho-analysis, appears to believe. By determinism we mean that every action and thought is the infallible result of a series of previous actions and thoughts and that there is no free will. In the first place Freud's belief or otherwise in this matter does not in any way affect the main principles of psycho-analysis, but is purely personal to himself, and were it proved to be a fact that there is no free will, although it would certainly interfere with some people's religious beliefs, it would not be likely, as many infer, to alter in the slightest the general conduct of humanity nor make men more inclined to be criminal, for the simple reason that living gregariously as they do the majority of their codes of conduct are based upon mutual convenience and happiness; and if a man said: " I have no free will; therefore there is nothing to prevent me from being a thief and I cannot help it if I am one," he would nevertheless probably not become a thief because of the actions which he has performed from childhood in accordance with his code and environment, which would force him to conform to their teaching, for in that way alone would he gain the greatest benefit. Thieves would still be thieves; the honest man would remain honest. But personally, I do not accept the theory of determinism as fully proved, not because if it were true I should be averse from finding it to be true, but because so far Freud's evidence to my mind is insufficient and, in fact, does not *prove* it.   Freud's observations do indeed show that the majority of our actions are ruled by previous events, environment, etc., but in some measure this was already known to everybody.   If we desire to walk from one room to the other we practically do not use free will: there is no debate on the matter: in the next room food is prepared for us; we are hungry, we feed, in much the same way as the bird picks up its worm when it is hungry, and further back, the earth-worm burrows through the ground or the unicellular amœba without brain or nerve system by some subtle force spreads itself round its food and absorbs it. ⸱ When we walk to the station in the morning our legs move mechanically; we do not use our *free* will with a definite active thought: one leg must be placed before the other in order to progress in the desired direction.   So throughout the day, habit, the result of past actions or thought, rules at least 99 per cent. of our lives. This we know, but it does not prove that on occasion we have no free will. ⸱ Freud has taken us a step further in thus understanding that determinism is at the basis of the majority of actions in our lives; he shows that if a man is asked to think of a number, on analysis the reason why he thought of that number is fairly easily found, and that no other number could possibly have been chosen under the circumstances. He says that when a man puts the wrong key into the latch of his front-door in an absent-minded manner that he could not possibly have done otherwise: that this action is the result of thoughts which have been stirred by other actions outside his control during the day. In the same way when we mentioned in the first chapter that a house surgeon had left his light burning with the unconscious motive of deceiving his chief we demonstrated that the action was determined for him and that he could not possibly have done otherwise.

Freud in his book on the " Psychopathology of Everyday Life " and in other works gives many convincing examples that much in our character, that many of our actions evil and good are quite beyond our control at any given moment. But there is one thing that appears to have been overlooked, and that is, *that in all the examples given one could not conceivably utilise free will in any case.* If I ask you to think of a number what opportunity do you get of using your will power? If you put the wrong latch-key into the door by accident, have you made any effort to use will power ? When a patient is suffering from hysteria due to repressions of various kinds, in that particular matter *the will power has already been lost.* When a chronic alcoholic is unable to cease from drinking it is what we may term the hysterical counter-will that is working, or, if you like, determinism. The will has no opportunity of working then. In all the examples which Freud gives one discovers on careful investigation that for some reason or another there is no opportunity for the use of free will. I am not setting out here to prove that free will exists ; I have no evidence on the matter : but I am setting out to show that the evidence already gathered does not prove its non-existence, but merely that *in the majority* of our thoughts we have neither the opportunity to use, nor do we use any will. When determinism does rule we may liken it physically to this : a patient sits down and crosses one leg over the other and leaves his leg hanging free. On tapping him smartly beneath the patella the foot will kick ; the knee jerk has been elicited. If this is done fifty times the result will be the same fifty times. There is movement of the leg, but this movement is predetermined. · On the other hand this does not prove that no other movement of the leg is possible. Under the conditions just given the man's will, or the freedom of the leg, is merely *eliminated during that period*. Or again, we may liken it to a locomotive standing at the top of a hill; if the brake be taken off, the locomotive will run down the hill, and will do it every time : but this will not prove that did somebody happen to put the brake on half-way down the hill the engine would then cease to move. Yet again, the actions which we may ascribe to our will are no doubt strictly limited by other determined conditions. The man on the engine may run it backwards or forwards, but only within the very much prescribed limits which the rails allow. Therefore we may accept this much determinism, that if there be free will, its action is infrequent, and its capabilities are strictly circumscribed by determinism.

꜀ A third objection to psycho-analysis is equally fallacious with those already quoted. It is, that it is dangerous to show people what evil things exist within them ; for by showing a man that he has, say, the tendency of a thief, you may make him a thief, by showing him that he has sexually perverted wishes in his unconscious you may make him a sexual pervert. As a matter of fact the practice of psycho-analysis has already proved by result that not only is this

.T

not the case, but that in every instance the analysed person is left stronger, more self-reliant and better from every point of view. But a moment's thought would show that if a man's disgust of thieving or of sexual perversion be so great that he has had the power to banish the tendency completely from his conscious mind, he would certainly have enough of a feeling of disgust and enough power to prevent him from falling into such errors consciously, when he is fortified by his knowledge of the unconscious in that direction.

Psycho-analysis never gives a man a tendency towards anything at all ; it merely reveals to his conscious mind the tendencies which he already possesses and the force of these tendencies is lessened thereby. Added to this is the fact that he is no longer wasting psychic energy in an unconscious and fruitless conflict which he does not understand, but can now direct his energy in a conscious and fully controlled manner.

CHAPTER XIV

The Scope of Psycho-Analysis

In considering the field which psycho-analysis covers and may cover in the future one has an enormous scope, which one must unfortunately for the moment endeavour to restrict, in so far as the present discussion is concerned.

Firstly, and of primary importance to readers of this book, we have the psycho-therapeutic field. Here we are able to cure the many hysterias and neuroses which have already been discussed at some length in previous chapters; added to these we have many conditions not so commonly recognised as psychoneurotic in origin —such for instance as kleptomania, where the kleptomaniac has exactly the same infantile repressions as the collector of stamps or pottery. It is true that one steals and the other buys, but the underlying psychic condition, the underlying relentless driving force is exactly the same, and, though the kleptomaniac cannot be cured by long terms of imprisonment yet he or she in many instances may be readily cured by psycho-analysis. The same applies to pyromania where we have an obsessional desire for fire, whether it be satisfied by setting fire to a haystack or to a large building. Many a person is imprisoned for this who is no more responsible for it than a man obsessed with the idea that he must tread on the cracks between the paving-stones. Again, drug habits, and in many instances alchoholism are traceable to the same source—infantile repressions, parental complexes and so forth, and what is more important, are curable by the same means, *viz.* :—psycho-analysis. This does not of course apply to every case, because habit, apart from environment, has in many instances played a part which persists in spite of any transformation which one is able to effect by analysis ; but certainly in young adults most of the obsessions referred to, which are not generally classed as neuroses, are curable by its means. We have dealt at so great length on the cure of psycho-neuroses in the earlier part of this book that it is not necessary to labour the point further here.

A second field which is now being entered upon very seriously by many educationalists is that of the psycho-analysis of children. Here we not only learn by the analysis of the child's mind how sometimes terrible mistakes are being made in its environment and upbringing but we are able to some extent to eradicate bad traits, even those of a trifling nature so often found in children such as temper, laziness, lying (a true psycho-neurotic condition) stealing, and other tendencies which so often render the parents thoroughly miserable. The energy expended on these can be frequently turned into the higher channels of sublimation by psychoanalysis of the child's mind. Pfister, and other analysts, have in part the honour of having organised this kind of work in Switzerland as a part of the education of children. Other countries are taking the matter up, though slowly, and it will probably be some time before its enormous educational value is realised.

Apart from the actual analysis of children we have perhaps a greater field still in adopting prophylactic measures as the result of psychoanalysis. Thus even in the short scope of this book we have disclosed several important points. Excessive kissing and physical signs of affection on the part of parents and others should be avoided from infancy. Children should not be encouraged to show off before strangers, nor to expose themselves for admiration, *e.g.*, in the bath, on every possible occasion, as is so often the case. Children of both sexes should be taught naturally and simply the true facts of sex—for plants, animals and men, and should not be taught to view them with disgust, but with a sane idea of control of appetite. Children whether of the same or the opposite sex should not be allowed to share bedrooms and more particularly beds with other children (nor with their parents) even at the age of two years. Children of both sexes should be brought up on identical lines, and an *artificial* differentiation in games, clothing and habits should not be forced upon them; indeed, it would be better for humanity if the artificial differentiation did not even come at puberty. Constipation in children stimulates the anal-erotic impulses, but it should not be treated by means of enemas. Children should not be allowed artificial teats to suck as it stimulates the labial-erotic and possibly the masturbatory impulses. On the other hand physical punishment in young children is liable to be very harmful in stimulating the aggressive, sadistic and masochistic impulses; and children should under no circumstances be frightened by bogies, policemen, and so forth.

❡ A third, and perhaps in some ways an even greater field where psycho-analysis is and will be of increasing importance is in its influence on the everyday life of mankind. Already the science has confirmed irrefutably some of the vague suppositions which many had felt rather than expressed in words as regards the relationship of the sexes, and it will no doubt be a guide in future in the evolution of civilisation. This is a point upon which I, perhaps, as a physician should not in this book lay too much stress ; nevertheless, as a help to those who are reading it rather from the broader point of view of sociology than from that of pure medical treatment, it may be well to touch on one of the points that obviously arise. We know that of recent years, for instance, the question of women's votes, and even more recently, of women's equality of pay with men have come to the forefront, but these when viewed from the point of psychoanalysis are merely straws in the wind. What we find underlying this is the greatest paradox in life. We find a civilised world in which the code, the teaching, the religion says that sexual matters shall be taboo, shall be relegated to the background, shall be driven from the mind as far as possible, and so forth ; yet this same world devotes nine-tenths of its energy to increasing the attraction between the sexes, the pleasure to be obtained by their intercourse, and in fact, by adding as much *artificial* differentiation over and above that which nature has itself bestowed as is humanly possible, with the appalling result that, while it teaches morality it breeds the most potent forms of perversion and immorality as fast as it can. It is not desirable to go into details here ; one might devote a

volume to the subject. Let us take a few of the
simplest distinctions made between the sexes.
There is no objective reason, saving that of
propagation of the species, why a male should
be addressed as Mr. and a female as Miss, why
male names should be of one type and female
names of another. The postman would find as
easily the owner of an initial and an address,
or at the utmost two initials. *It is merely that
we are striving at the first and earliest opportunity to make a differentiation and to keep it
in mind!* At our dinner parties again, there
is no essential intellectual reason why male and
female should be alternated round the table.
From the highest point of view, or, if you like,
from the most interesting point of view, any
two persons who have a common topic of conversation should sit next to one another, irrespective of sex, though this sex, it will be observed, is thrust upon them willy nilly. One
often notices too, how what is termed courtesy
towards the weaker sex is not courtesy but
etiquette, and is really something quite apart
from true unselfishness. For instance I have
many times seen a man, possibly suffering from
varicose veins or some other disability, offer
his seat in a tram to a woman—perhaps a girl—
in the bloom of health, carrying a hockey stick,
and obviously suffering from no disability at

the moment. His real attitude is exemplified, however, when the woman less trammelled than some, politely refuses to recognise a disability by taking the offered seat. It will often then be observed that the man also refuses to sit down, and indeed may become quite angry. His real concern is not that the woman is standing, but for his position in the eyes of the other passengers and even much more so for the position of his sex as a superior type, which can afford to give away small mercies. As a matter of fact, it is obvious to any psycho-analyst, or indeed to anyone who has nullified his infantile repressions and early associations by conscious self-examination, that real chivalry is not a question of such minor matters as what one sex gives to another, but what youth gives to age or strength to weakness irrespective of sex ; and one does not wonder that some women who have the cause of their sex at heart feel insulted by the manner in which they are treated in these and similar respects, for it is because they realise intuiti ely rather than consciously that there is something unpleasant in the unconscious that is the cause of the play-acting.

When we look round we realise that a very large number of our shops, our habits, our very lives indeed are devoted to an exhibition of the charms of woman. They may appeal to the hetero-sexual, the homo-sexual or the auto-sexual, and in most cases, as will be understood by those who have read the earlier chapters of this book, they certainly involve infantile sexual perversions, though it is true that these perversions are not generally recognised as such, for the very simple reason that no person easily recognises his own complexes ; in those things in which he deceives himself he is deceived by others. There is no doubt that those who have had what may be called " The Women's Movement " at heart have seen something of this, and one is inclined to prophecy that these same people or their descendents will see to it that moral education takes such steps and makes such changes as to ensure that the woman of the future is not differentiated from the man either as regards, clothing, business remuneration or anything else artificial. They will realise that the extra energy of sex is not to be *displaced* as it is at present, but should be *sublimated* ; that there will always remain enough of unsublimated sex to propagate the species and carry on the race to yet higher ideals. One may quote from the women's pages of our evening newspapers or call attention to clothing exhibited in many of our shops, to show that where such points as I have mentioned are so obvious that the least intelligent would see their truth. It is where the exaggeration is not so great and where the mind has become accustomed to a certain condition of things, that the truth is not readily recognised. For instance, a woman whose exhibition tendency is not great, will decry a decolleté neck of say, six inches all round; and possibly a woman wearing such a decolleté neck will decry a woman wearing a frock which leaves the whole of the back bare. In each case the principle remains the same; it is merely a question of degree, and it is only by analysis (not necessarily by an analyst, but sometimes by self-analysis alone,) that the fact of these most unpleasant home truths is borne in upon one.

In these facts we may also see at least one of the reasons why so few women attain to great-ness in either the sciences or arts, etc. It is not that they lack intellect, they often have the same powers of understanding as their brothers. It is that they lack psychic energy behind their non-erotic ideas. *So much of their energy is wasted on displaced erotic ideas, that they have not sufficient energy left for the sublimated forms to compete with the sublimated energy of men.* It is true, men's eroticism is more open and less displaced, and therefore more noticeable to the community, but it is in fact women who devote the greatest percentage of psychic energy to erotic matters. And until women aim more at sublimation and less at displacement, they are not likely to gain the equality to which they are entitled, in fact—the equality in work and in achievement, which, for instance the horse and the mare already possess.

For this reason one strongly recommends women who intend to become psycho-analysts to be analysed themselves, in the first instance by a man—because I have noticed in one or two women analysts whom I know personally that they still possess many of their complexes in the unconscious condition, and are therefore unable to analyse them in others. On this account, I have on one or two occasions had to re-analyse a woman patient who had failed to recognise complexes which her analyst also possessed. It arises of course from the fact that women have so much more repressed material, and so much greater resistance than the normally educated man.

We pride ourselves on being civilised, and having thrust the primitive barbarian far from us, but in fact our evolution has but reached a halfway house, and in many respects we are more perverted than some of the South Sea islanders, because we have taken much of the energy which they must still devote to self-preservation and side-tracked it into erotic channels.

Not that this phase through which humanity has passed in the last few thousand years has been without its value in evolution. Ego-centricity, selfishness, exaggerated and artificial sex differences have all contributed to the hastening of intellectual evolution.

The first great instinct necessary for physical evolution was that of self-preservation. When such a type as man was produced, self-preservation in its primordial sense called for less energy and that energy was placed elsewhere. Selfishness, self-gratification, became the ruling instinct, and intellect was developed out of it. Self-gratification said: " I want more comcomfort," and a bed was invented; "I want yet more comfort" and a motor car resulted. The intellect was used and trained by this ego-centric instinct of which artificial sex differentiation was a part on account of the interaction of the erotic instinct.

But now that this has been accomplished, the ego-centric impulses lose much of their communal value, a higher or psychic development is in progress, and as self-preservation instincts have become but trivial in man, so these other ego-centric instincts are being undermined, and this is part of the training of psychic evolution. *Sublimation, not displacement, is the end in view.*

As for the psychic energy itself, whence it

comes and what it is we have no evidence. It may be that it is ultimately a transformation of physical energy. We have not even evidence that we derive it from our food; for all we know it may come from outside, for it is obvious in the experiments in telepathy I described in the first chapter that it *can* pass between individuals through space, without contact. There are many and varied speculations, and I only mention them here as a warning against dogmatism. Some psycho-analysts have assumed that no energy can come except from the food we eat. It may be so; but there is no evidence. Negative evidence is not evidence at all; the only way to progress is to keep an open mind; and at present the ultimate source of psychic energy is—*nescio*.

INDEX

A.

Abreaction, 106, 191
Actual Neuroses, 149
Aggression, 43
Aggression, in compulsion neurosis, 174
Agoraphobia, 165
Alcoholism, 23
Alcoholism, in compulsion neurosis, 179
Alcoholism in exhibitionism, 102
Alcoholism in homosexuality, 102
Alcoholism in narcissism, 102
Anal Eroticism, 52, 68, 90, 91
Anal Eroticism and dreams, 142
Anal Eroticism in folie du doute, 177
Analysis of dreams, 134
Anus, 50
Anxiety Hysteria, 150, 161
Anxiety Hysteria, sexual disturbance in, 161
Anxiety Hysteria, signs and symptoms, 161
Anxiety Neuroses, 149, 184
Anxiety Neuroses, breathing in, 189
Anxiety Neuroses, causes of, 185
Anxiety Neuroses, characteristics of, 186
Anxiety Neuroses, mechanism of, 185
Anxiety Neuroses, treatment of, 190
Artificial sex differentiation, 59 87, 282, 283
Association, 1, 6, 10
Association method, 198
Association method, types of reaction, 205
Automatic writing, 179, 229

Automatic writing, analysis of, 241
Automatic writing, example of, 236
Autosexuality, 36, 39
Autosexuality in women, 50

B.

Beauty, 57, 154
Bisexuality, 37, 44, 52, 56, 87. 91
Blood-pressure in anxiety neurosis, 189, 193
Blood-pressure in neurasthenia, 195
Breathing in anxiety neuroses, 189

C.

Censor, 73, 129, 136
Censor, when careless, 142
Character, formation of, 75
Chemio-taxis, 48
Child, analysis of, 280
Child, desires unrepressed, 125
Child, dreams of, 128
Child, education of, 27, 280
Child, eldest, 104
Child, only, 104, 170
Child, phantasies, 126, 141
Claustrophobia, 165
Cloacal Eroticism, 88
Coitus interruptus, 186
Coitus reservatus, 186
Complex, 11, 54, 75
Complex, Electra, 77
Complex, Homosexual, 82
Complex, "Intelligence," 206
Complex, Narcissistic, 97
Complex, Nuclear, 77
Complex, Œdipus, 77

INDEX